Autobiographical Notes of Louis A. Gottschalk

AUTOBIOGRAPHICAL NOTES OF LOUIS A. GOTTSCHALK

LOUIS A. GOTTSCHALK

Nova Science Publishers, Inc.
New York

For permission to use material from this book please contact us:
Telephone 631-231-7269; Fax 631-231-8175
Web Site: http://www.novapublishers.com

LIBRARY OF CONGRESS CATALOGING-IN-PUBLICATION DATA

Gottschalk, Louis A. (Louis August), 1916-
Autobiographical notes of Louis A. Gottschalk / Louis A. Gottschalk.
p. cm.
Includes index.
ISBN-13: - 978- 1-60021-429-5
ISBN -10 – 1-60021-429-0
1. Gottschalk, Louis A. (Louis August), 1916- . 2. Psychiatrists --United States--Biography. I. Title.
[DNLM: 1. Gottschalk, Louis A. (Louis August), 1916- . 2. Psychiatry--United States--Biography. WZ 100 G6867 2006]
RC438.6.G68A3 2006
616.890092--dc22
[B]

2006028520

Published by Nova Science Publishers, Inc. ✦ New York

CONTENTS

AUTOBIOGRAPHICAL REFLECTIONS

MEMORIES

Early Memories

The earliest memory I ever had, which came to me in a dream during my personal (training) psychoanalysis with Dr. George Mohr, M.D. (Dean of the Institute for Psychoanalysis in Chicago during 1947) was of myself as a little baby climbing some huge stairs from the first floor of a house to the second floor. As this baby, I was crawling up these stairs looking for my mother. On a landing between the first and second floors there were some sketches on the wall facing me. I stared at them for a while, very colorful I thought, maybe monsters, and I kept on climbing these huge stairs. Finally, I got to a place that looked like a kitchen (on the second floor), and in that kitchen I saw my mother and my father talking and someone else. I cannot say who it was. I was very glad to find my mother. For - several years, thereafter, whenever I voluntarily evoked that dream-scene, tears would come to my eyes, and I would unexpectedly feel very sad.

Sometime later, I asked my mother whether there was a place in St. Louis where our family lived that had a kitchen on the second floor, for I could not recall any other place we lived that had a kitchen in such a location. Maybe it was the house on 3409 Lucas Avenue in St. Louis, I reflected, where my parents lived for a while with uncle Louis and aunt Annie and my maternal grandparents. My mother said there was, indeed, a kitchen on the second floor. I asked her if there were some paintings on the wall on the landing between the first and second floor, and she said that there were, paintings of "monsters" that my father had made. I do not have any other early memories about the Lucas Avenue residence, but I do remember the house from the outside, for I remember seeing it many times when I was older. My parents would point it out to me as they drove by it.

I was born on August 26, 1916, and I estimated that I was less than 1 year of age when I had that experience depicted in my dream. After reviewing the excellent Mutrux biographical monograph written by Philippe Mutrux a cousin to determine whether it would provide any pertinent information for my recollections, I discovered that my maternal grandfather (Jules Auguste Mutrux) was born on December 02,1844, and he died on January 10, 1917. My mother must have been grieving about her father's (my maternal grandfather) passing away. And I was only about 4.5 months of age at that time. That seems to me to be a very early memory involving details of a place and of emotions, and there is convincing evidence that the memory was a valid one.

Furthermore, I learned from cousin Philip's monograph (See footnote on page 2) that the Gottschalks did, indeed, live with the Mutrux family, both maternal grandparents, uncle Louis and aunt Annie, and the children they had at that time, namely, Edward, Robert, and John (Jean) in that Lucas Avenue residence. (Philip gives these names in French spellings, probably because as children we were all required to speak French, especially to my mother and when visiting the Mutrux family in Clayton, Missouri.)

The Gottschalks and the Mutruxes

I was the third of four sons by my parents. Max Jules, my oldest brother was born on December 14, 1909; Edmond was born on July 17, 1913; I was born on August 26, 1916; and Charles was born on March 15, 1919 (I learned that Charlie had not yet been born while we Gottschalks lived in the Lucas Avenue dwelling.)

Uncle Louis and aunt Annie had lots of children, a total of 12, and I think that about the time the Mutrux's lived at the Lucas Avenue residence, they must have had three of the first children, as I said before the oldest being Edward and the next being Robert and the next John ("Jean" according to Philip's spelling.).

Both my father and uncle Louis were artists at the time and one or both of them could have been involved with the paintings on the stairway wall.

My father went to the law school at the University of Missouri at Columbus, Missouri (His father and his uncle were both lawyers), and after finishing law school, he decided he did not want to be a lawyer. When I asked my father, how come, he said that there was lots of music in his home. His father was a singer as well as a lawyer. He and his brother (Victor Hugo Gottschalk) had piano and violin lessons. And, I cannot resist mentioning it, fisticuffs lessons. I do not know why. (Maybe that is one of the reasons he took us boys to boxing and prize fight shows.) He wanted to be a musician, composer, and artist. And he married Kelmie Mutrux, my mother, who played the piano*. And uncle Louis married Ann Von der Ahe, who also played the piano.*

"Kelmie became the wife of Max Gottschalk several years after our parents married. Max, an artist and musician, was involved in our parent's meeting (probably in 1900). Maman, was a gifted pianist. She won awards, gave concerts and played with Max and other musicians. Kelmie also played piano and gave lessons. Philippe, Suzette, and Louise were among her pupils."

"The Gottschalks lived at 6000 Waterman Avenue during the years we knew them. When Max and Kelmie married and during the time Jules Max "Buzzie", Edmond Fredric and Louis Auguste were born, they lived at 3409 Lucas Avenue near Grand Avenue in St. Louis, in a house owned by Jules Auguste and Louise Berney, parents of Papa and Kelmie. Our parents also lived there during the time Edouard Jules, Robert Henri, and Jean Louis were born. Then they moved to 6002 Waterman Avenue. My earliest memories of my cousins are of the period after they had left Lucas and were living at 7416 Washington Avenue in University City.

---

* Excerpted from Biography of Louis Eugene Mutrux and La Famille by Philippe G. Mutrux (unpublished document), pp. 20-22.

Aunt Kelmie was encouraging us (Philippe, Ernest, Edmond, and Louis) to prepare our lunch in the side yard of their house, the menu being canned beans and frankfurters cooked on a grill over a little campfire. This was the occasion of the "Boston Cooking Club" which never met again. We met our cousins occasionally at which time we would compete at making pencil drawings. An amusing occurrence from this period was when their colored maid was terrified on seeing "strange" gloves hanging on the clothesline, thinking they belonged to some weird simian-like animal or person. These "gloves" were simply uncle Max's socks which were made with articulated toes.

"Another episode was uncle Max driving up to the Grand Central Theatre in his soft-top Oldsmobile with a live chicken clutching to the top. Max was a "dandy" affecting spats, a monocle and a cane."

"We got along well with our Gottschalk cousins (which wasn't the case with some of our other cousins). We were in awe of uncle Max; whereas, aunt Kelmie seemed quiet, placid, and self-effacing. Our swimming pool was an important factor in our relationship with the Gottschalks. Many a summer afternoon, uncle Max would bring interesting people along with his own family. There were musicians, singers, artists, and on one occasion he brought along an aviator (a rare bird in the mid-1920s). Some of the guests included Harvey Enders, a composer-singer-arranger; Max Steindel, a cellist; the Gusicoff brothers, violinists; and Richard Miller, an artist...."

"In the early years Buzzie stood out as the most creative and interesting cousin. He was interested in many fields, such as, manufacturing wooden bows and arrows, kites and kite flying, and as a pianist, he played Gershwin, and Eric Satie. He experimented with electronic music, and he owned and drove exotic racing cars. Edmond, Louis, and Charles were around but in the background in those days. Via the Gottschalks we met people interested in art, music, and culture in general. This enriched our lives significantly, and they deserve our thanks. Uncle Max was the Impresario running the show and although autocratic, argumentative, domineering and vain, he was also humorous, imaginative, witty, and energetic. They were involved with Papa in some real estate investments. The six-family apartment building at 6000 Waterman Avenue, which they owned and lived in for many years, was designed and built by Papa. There were other properties co-owned by both parties; however, details are missing. Papa at one time was the creator and president of four real estate corporations. The other stockholders were friends, relatives and local people of Swiss extraction. Uncle Max played violin with the Saint Louis Symphony and the Municipal Opera in Forest Park. He also organized various string quartets and trios. He had hopes of becoming president of the local Musicians Union, but was probably too controversial and domineering. He was a great conversationalist refusing to allow the hint of 'Political Correction' to hinder his flow of thought."

"In 1924 the Gottschalks went to Europe. Louis Gottschalk has written a biography entitled 'Memoirs of my Mother' in which he describes many details of the trip as well as the Lucas Avenue days until March 8, 1953 when aunt Kelmie died."

"Our family went to Switzerland the following year returning in 1926."

Leaving the details cited in the document of my cousin Phil and returning to my own recollections, I remember my Uncle Louis going with a mutual friend (Richard Miller) of my father and himself to Paris, France to study art. Richard Miller did become a famous artist, and I have a portrait of my paternal grandfather and my father that Richard Miller painted (unsigned) and a painting of my paternal grandmother that Richard Miller's sister (Viola

Miller) painted. The painting of my paternal grandmother (not signed) and my paternal grandfather are interesting in many ways, but I never knew them personally, for they died before I was born. But I do have a small picturesque painting of a scene in France, signed by Viola Miller and dated 1913. As a boy, I met both Richard Miller and Viola Miller. My father had many artist and musician friends. Father played first violin in the St. Louis Symphony; he had a string quartet which played for wealthy sponsors. He also composed much music. And for a while he wrote music and art critiques for the St. Louis Post Dispatch.

When uncle Louis returned to St. Louis from his studies and trips to Switzerland and France, he tried to make a living as an artist and could not do so, I am told. So he became a builder and an architect, and built many properties, residences and apartments, with the help of his many children, some of whom became architects and engineers. Uncle Louis converted to the Catholic Apostolic faith while he was in France, and he became very devoted to that faith giving weekly readings and services to his children (all in French) at his residence and ten-acre farm on Dielman Road in Clayton, Missouri. As a little six-year-old boy, temporarily living with the Mutrux family and recuperating from the stress reactions of a tonsillectomy, adenoidectomy, and circumcision operation (all on the same day) at the Missouri Baptist Hospital—by arrangement of my dear mother and dear aunt Annie—I convalesced at the Mutrux farm for a week or so and slept with a bunch of Mutrux children. I recall that I attended and heard uncle Louis do his religious readings to his family (and me), all in French. Let me now get back to my other earlier memories.

I was quite a thumb sucker as a child. I remember our family living at 7416 Washington in University City, Missouri. In the back yard we raised chickens, and I was fascinated by them. Once, to my surprise, a rooster flew up at me and pecked me on the face leaving a little scar. Papa explained to us boys that roosters sometimes do not like others in the hen house yard, even if they are only collecting eggs. And I do clearly remember papa cutting off a chicken's head with an ax when the chicken was going to become a meal. I watched and wondered at the severed head as its beak opened and closed a few times.

Going back to the thumb sucking, I remember mother putting some reddish powder on both my thumbs, which was bitter and did not taste very good. I found out that if I sucked through the bitter stuff, I could suck my thumb comfortably. I got the idea then that with my own children and after some child psychoanalytic training, maybe thumb sucking was not so bad (a lingering need for attachment to the mother and her breast) and that there is considerable genetic difference in the urge to suck thumbs (or twirl one's hair, as girls often do). (Having got some information from Philippe's Mutrux family biography, now I wonder whether that little baby crawling up those stairs was looking for its mother to be close to her and to suckle on her breasts. Maybe that was a contributor to my persistent thumb sucking.) Anyway, another early memory while living at 7416 Washington, I do remember sucking through the bitter red stuff. Sometime along the way—around age 4 or so--I stopped thumb sucking, rather gradually.

I do remember a pretty girl neighbor who lived across the street; her name was Cynthia. She invited me to a birthday party. I remember what she looked like; she had curly hair and wore dresses. We Gottschalk children were all boys and wore shorts and long pants. At that age I never wondered what her genital organs were like; I rather assumed they were like what we boys and my papa had.

I remember my maternal grandmother. She usually wore black clothes, and always spoke French to us. She was very loving and she would, on some occasions, give us little pieces (about ½ centimeter in length) of cylindrical licorice, which tasted very good. (Now I reflect that her husband had died, Jules Auguste Mutrux by name, and that is why she wore black). I have photographs of my maternal grandmother and paternal grandmother together; this must have been at a time when we lived at the Lucas Avenue address in St. Louis.

Several years later, I remember my mother being sad, and she told us boys that our grandmother had died. (I learned later as an adult that she died of colon cancer in 1925. According to Philip's monograph, she lived with us at 7416 Washington. There was a funeral for grandmother Mutrux (Louise was her first name, Philip says). All the Mutrux family and other relatives and we Gottschalks got together for the funeral service. My memory of those events was that it was a happy one---all the family got together, people prayed, and later we had a lot of good food. Oh yes, the Notts were there: Grandaunt Marie, and her offspring, Marie, Minerva and Charles, and they all spoke French. I do remember their house. It was nice and smelled of tobacco. And Marie and Minerva fussed over us little boys.

Adventures Abroad

Well, in 1924 my father made some money from a lot he sold in St. Louis. I think it was $10,000.00 (I am sure that was a lot of money in the 1920's). My parents were not rich. After all, father was a musician and artist and mother gave piano lessons. But they must have inherited some money from my father's parents and my mother's parents, which had enabled them to buy the house in University City, Missouri. And papa decided he should blow the money. (Good for him! He was an adventurer and good, but strict with his offspring.) He wanted all of us to go to Europe and visit our relatives—his relatives in Germany and mother's relatives in Switzerland and France. My father also arranged to go to Provincetown, Rhode Island where he was going to do some art work. My mother's assignment was to take us four boys to Switzerland, first to Paris, France via the ocean liner, The President Harding, and then eventually to Lausanne, Geneva, Yverdon, Orges, Trecovagnes, and other towns where mother's relatives lived. She had corresponded with many of them for years

I was seven years old, and those were fun times with my mother and four brothers. And on an ocean liner! I can recall many of the details, especially visually, waiting for the ship to take off in the New York harbor, tugboats pulling us, the ship getting underway, the ship rocking a bit. We boys were fascinated by everything on deck, the life boats, the fog horns, the ventilators. We were gently reprimanded for trying to climb up into them and hanging on them. It was an exciting experience. It prepared us for our return voyage from France to New York, this time with papa, on the Leviathan, a very large ship at that time. But details of that come later.

In Paris, France, I can clearly visualize the hotel room where mother booked us. She left all four of us in the room for a while and went to phone my father in Provincetown and make travel arrangements to go by rail to Geneva, Switzerland. We boys waited and played in the room and got a great idea. Play hide and seek! The clever idea was to have one of us kids hide in a bureau drawer, selecting one several drawers up. And I was one of the kids who was to hide in the drawer. When my older brothers pulled out the drawer, I climbed up the outside of the chiffoniere to do so. As I did, the whole chiffoniere, which had a very large mirror in the front of it, fell forward and the glass mirror shattered. We just could not think of a way to put the pieces of mirror together before mother returned to the hotel room. When mother came back to the hotel room, she was—of course—astounded. She asked how it happened, and we told her. She went downstairs and called the concierge who came up to look at the mess.

Shamefacedly, we boys watched the transaction that took place, all communications in French, between mother and the hotel manager. And we saw mother giving the gentleman some travelers' checks. The astounding detail about this memory is that mother never upbraided us about the event. We boys, separately or jointly, got into other little problems and mischief, I should admit. And she took them in her stride, calmly. There is no doubt in my mind that this mother of ours absolutely loved boys. She was tolerant, patient, forgiving, instructive, helpful, sympathetic, empathic. She paid attention to our individual differences and tried to accommodate our different personalities. She was the same way with my father, patient, helpful, and, yes, accommodating. Now I realize, as a professor and practicing neuropsychiatrist, how fortunate we were to have had such a mother (and such a father). (The parents of many of the patients I see—children and adults—hardly match her motherly and feminine virtues and personality.)

Well, we went on by train to Lausanne, and we ended up at what seemed to me like a large, tall building on Lac Leman. It had an elevator, and we had an apartment on one of the upper floors. We boys were encouraged to walk on the streets of Lausanne and explore it while mother went shopping. There were some children rolling hoops and they were dressed in peculiar clothes, not pants or shorts. And going by one house on the street, some children yelled at us in words we could not understand. And we yelled back at them. There were three of them, and they had long hair and something like skirts and not pants or shorts. Pretty soon we all started hollering at each other. They looked so strange and funny. And I guess we looked odd to them. Our mother came along, and she went into the courtyard of the house and their mother came out. And the two women began to talk. It turned out that the children were of German-Swiss ethnicity, they were speaking German to us, and they could also speak French, but not English. My brothers and I started speaking French to them and they spoke French to us. And we all became friends, and they even showed us their toys and let us play with them. And they taught us to play with and roll hoops with them. What a lesson in communication and the healing effect of understandable verbal messages!

The voyage back to the United States on the Leviathon (a big ocean liner in those days) was memorable. We four boys had become old hands at this sort of travel. We were well behaved, and we traveled in Tourist Class, which was not the same as First Class, but it seemed elegant to us. We did learn that we were not supposed to venture into the First Class portion of the ship. And papa was on this ocean voyage with us back to the United States, which probably made the child care portion easier for mother, but that is just a guess, for we had no knowledge about parental responsibilities.

New York, New York

We learned as we neared New York City that papa was going to stay in New York. In fact, the whole Gottschalk family was going to do so, because papa was going to work for the Wurlitzer Company as an appraiser and seller of fine violins and other stringed instruments. Father was an expert in this area, and I can remember books on fine violins I saw in our apartment in New York, New York (690 Riverside Drive), and later came across in our apartment in St. Louis, Missouri (6000 Waterman Avenue).

In New York City, I remember our parents exploring the school system, even a private school, and they decided we would go to the public school. The public school was acceptable. About the time I was going there I lost my two front teeth, and when I talked I tended to lisp. One day I was called on to recite in class, and I got up and said whatever I had to say in response to the teacher's request. To my surprise, the other students laughed at what I said or how I said it—apparently because I lisped somewhat. The teacher told the students to stop laughing and took me out in the school hall with her. "Louis, why did you talk that way?" she asked. "I couldn't help it, because my two front teeth came out" I said, pointing to where they had been. She abruptly came up to me and slapped me in the face over my mouth and told me to come back in the classroom and be quiet. Thereafter, I believe I had a, perhaps, mild school phobia. For sometimes I would have a stomach ache after breakfast, and I would complain to my mother. She would let me stay home and the next day or so, she would write a note, an excuse, saying "Louis did not feel well" yesterday or for whatever number of days I was absent. For many years after that, I used to wonder why I was often afraid to get up in front of class and recite, for I would get anxious. Not until many years later—after getting a Child Psychiatry residency at Michael Reese Hospital in Chicago and during my personal (training) psychoanalysis—did I put together that that New York school teacher's slapping me in the face, so unexpectedly, played a part in my mild school phohia. (I say "mild" because I really liked school, and I wanted to be able to recite and perform as well as my father, a fine musician, a great performer, and a great talker and conversationalist. Over the years in growing up, I sought to be in plays and performances, tolerating the stage fright and hoping it would go away if I did well. The psychodynamics of that methodology is referred to as over-compensation, namely, recurring attempts to overcome a problem by persistently doing the behavior or feared performance again and again (metaphorically, like practicing over and over again a difficult and challenging portion of piano music).

In New York City, we boys had fun. There was a "dumb waiter" in our apartment. We got the good idea of one of us getting into the "dumb waiter" and having a brother let us go up and down to look into other people's apartments. Our parents caught us doing that and told us not to do it again.

We lived close to the Hudson River (or a tributary of it right in the city) and we would go down to the river, watch the boats go by, throwing things in the water, and let ourselves get wet. One time a door-sized board with some tar paper on one side washed up on the beach. My brothers, Edmond and Charlie, said we could pretend it was a raft like Tom Sawyer and Huckelberry Finn. I got on the make-believe raft and my brothers pushed it out into the flowing river. That was fun, but the raft got into the current. I had no paddle, and what do you know? Soon I was about 100 feet away from the shore, and the raft kept going out farther. My brothers spoke to some men working on nearby freight trains, switching them and so on, pointed at me on the raft, and asked whether they could help. Looking over the situation, I guess they could see that there was not much they could do; they had responsibilities with their jobs and the trains. The current carried me out farther and farther. I could swim but not well enough to get back to the shore. The trainmen phoned somebody, and a couple of men in a boat (Water policemen? I don't know) came next to the raft and rescued me and took me to the shore. Whew! Now that was a sort of exciting (and scary) adventure.

Well, we had lots of experiences in New York City. I will tell more of them. I know we went to Coney Island, but on the way—with papa driving—I fell asleep, so the rest of the family went to Coney Island, while I slept in the car for the rest of the evening. I cannot say I remember Coney Island.

Back to St. Louis, Missouri

But let us get back to St. Louis, and later I will tell more about our New York City experience.

In St. Louis, my parents owned a six-family apartment building, which had been designed and built by uncle Louis Mutrux and his construction company. The Mutrux family had lived next door at 6002 Waterman Avenue, a two-family dwelling, which uncle Louis had also designed and built before he moved his family to a ten-acre location on Dielman Road in Clayton, Missouri, definitely out in St. Louis County, where they had a cow, chickens, and they did some farming. More about that later perhaps, though my cousin Philip has written an excellent biographical monograph, which I will refer to from time to time.

While living at 6000 Waterman Avenue, we went to Hamilton Elementary School, from there to Ben Blewett Junior High School and then Soldan High School. If a student did well at Ben Blewett Junior High School (Latin was required and so was Mathematics, Science, English, Social Studies, History, and Physical Education), the student could do the middle school years in two, two and a half or three years. I was assigned to a two and one-half year group. I really did not know what difference that made.

I recall walking with my brothers to and from Ben Blewett from 6000 Waterman. Sometimes we got a ride from a parent, sometimes we took the street car, which cost 7 cents for a token and 10 cents otherwise.

I remember many details about our life during those days. Which ones to report is a question in my mind. Well, papa built a club house in our backyard for us kids that we could all use. That sparked a building urge in each one of us. We got wood scraps and boards from construction sites in the nearby neighborhood. I built a fairly good house with a two-way slooping roof. Charlie built one next to mine. And Edmond, not to be outdone by his little brothers, built what seemed at that time like a castle with a tower that had an inside ladder and a little flat roof with four glassless windows. What prompted us to do this building, as I reflect on the matter momentarily, were the building skills of my father, but also uncle Louis. When we visited the Mutrux farm in St. Louis County, we got into the habit of building tree houses in nearby trees. Sometimes this activity was competitive, for there was a pairing off of kids: Edmond, Philip, Ernest in one group and Louis, Charles, Oliver, Paul and George (the twins), and sometimes Richard (the youngest boy in the Mutrux family). I can evoke a visual memory of some of those tree houses—on neighboring trees with step ladders made by nailing foot-long boards onto the tree for steps. Carpentry ability was expected of each child. My father was skilled at this, and he was a wonderful woodcarver. Out of white pine, he carved different and distinctive swords for each of us boys. My oldest brother, Max Jules, became an expert, making marvelous bows and arrows that he sold, and later in life, he became known for his extraordinary furniture and as a famous industrial designer. If we younger kids were willing and obedient, he taught us and let us work on the furniture he designed and built for his company. John Mutrux grew to become a specialist in custom-building various kinds of furniture (chairs, desks, tables, and so forth). Like his older brothers (Edward and Robert), and younger ones (Philip, Ernest, Paul and George) they all went to

Washington University in St. Louis and obtained degrees in Architecture or Architectural Engineering.

Going to the University was a plan in my mind, but the 1929 economic depression, which extended into the early 1930's, made my going to a university to get a college education an unrealistic goal. After graduating from Soldan High School with a fairly good grade point average, I attended Hadley Vocational School (a public school in St. Louis) where I pursued vocational training in secretarial skills, bookkeeping, and a related curriculum. In secretarial training, I was taught typing, shorthand (the Gregg system), and in bookkeeping I was taught just that—namely, how to be a bookkeeper. (Wasn't Bob Cratchet a bookkeeper, the character in the Christmas story?) Some of the girls in these classes were really spectacular as speedy typists (the number of words typed per minute, the number of typing errors, and the corrected speed based on a formula that deducted a penalty from the total score) were fed back to us students so that we could compare ourselves to other pupils. The system had its virtues in matter of factly putting us all into a competitive framework, which could spur us all towards achieving the skill of typing. A similar system prevailed with respect to learning and accurately using Gregg shorthand. I attended Hadley Vocational School for one-half year (I graduated from Soldan High School December, 1934), and I completed the school at Hadley Vocational in June, 1935. I tried applying for jobs as a secretary, and I remember trying out for a position with a railroad office, where I was put to a stringent test, taking shorthand dictation from an office manager and typing some letters. I did as well as I could, but I did not get the job. I worked for a while at Krummenacher's Drug store, behind the cigarette and cigar counter for a while and behind the soda fountain. Mr. Krummenacher was a nice man; he and his family also lived near by us on Waterman Avenue. And I was sweet on his daughter, Helen, whom I dated for a while in those days. I could see her house from one of our apartment's windows. And I noted that this very pretty girl had other boy friends who would sometimes come by her house in an automobile. And I was jealous—yes I was. Her parents and her brother were cordial to me, and I was sometimes invited to their house to go on picnics with them and their friends. That was a good experience.

I finally got my first regular job at the First National Bank of St. Louis, which was located at Olive Street and Fifth Avenue. It was a very large bank in a building with many floors (7, I believe). My first job was handing out bank statements to customers who came to the bank for them. My boss there was Mr. Morris. Later I was upgraded to a position in the Personnel Department, where my job was to tabulate the attendance records of the employees and do various kinds of office work for my boss, Mr. Stauss. That is where I met one of my best friends in those days—Robert White—and later his brother, Bill White. Bob was a handsome tall, thin guy, the son of a banker who had died. He wrote interesting poetry, played the bassoon, was a very stylish dresser, and he bought fancy cars (like a Packard roadster) that he would take me riding in. His mother owned a restaurant near Irondale, Missouri, and he would take me out there, and we would do enjoyable things together. Later, I remember that he did a tour of duty during World War II in the Navy on an aircraft carrier, and I think that stressed him. I introduced him to a sometime girl friend of mine (Betty Chappel); he married her, they had children together, and later I learned that he died of a stroke. I have a photo of him, his brother, my brother Charlie, my father, my stepmother (Gladys, a former opera singer, who died of breast cancer, and who had a schizophrenic daughter), and myself taken at the Chase Hotel in St. Louis. They have all passed away, except me. Recalling these people and the mostly good times we had, evokes a bittersweet series of memories. I remember Bob White asked me why I was going to Washington University Medical School, and why did I want to be a neuropsychiatrist. At that time he was a successful businessman of some kind.

[On my computer at the Gottschalk Medical Plaza at UCI, I inserted some details regarding the death of my brother, Max Jules Gottschalk, born December 14, 1909 and died July 25, 2005 from a cerebral stroke. I am not going to write about that at this point.]

Well, I went to Washington University in St. Louis, Missouri, on a partial scholarship, starting there in September, 1936. Having taken some night school classes there, in Business Law and English, I had a few units of credits, and some good grades, which I believe helped me get the partial scholarship. I found going to the University very stimulating and exciting. I took English, French, History, Abnormal Psychology, Physiological Psychology and the Physiology of Sensation (under John Paul Nafe), History, Philosophy. Biology, General and Inorganic Chemistry, Organic Chemistry, Genetics, Qualitative and Quantitative Chemistry, Physiology, Experimental and Developmental Embryology, Art History, English Literature, Expository Writing, Physics, Premedical Physics, and other classes. I got interested in extracurricular activities. I tried out for the swimming team and later the fencing team. Because I turned out to be good in fencing foils, I was made the captain of the freshman fencing team. In swimming I was not bad as a free-style sprinter, but I never practiced, and I swam in a few relay matches. I wrote for the University newspaper, Student Life and also the University magazine, the Eliot. I also acted in some plays, I had some bit parts, and I even danced in a Musical Comedy. I did a love waltz in a white-tailed suit with a rather heavy girl (Hortense Holtgrewe) in a black dress, the daughter of a physician. By this time I aspired to go to Medical School, though I did not have the money. But thanks to Professor David Rioch who helped me get a Fellowshiop (Josiah Macy Foundation). I got some scholarship loan money and a Fellowship position in the Department of Neuropsychiatry (as it was called in those days, for it included both Psychiatry and Neurology), which paid $75.00/ month during the school year (nine months).

Working in the Department of Neuropsychiatry, which was headed by Dr John C. Whitehorn, M.D., I was assigned to work with Dr. Felix Deutsch, M.D. and his research fellow Dr. Richard Nadel, M.D. Those experiences got me into the new field of psychosomatic medicine, which was entirely new to me in those days. The head of Neurology was Dr. James O'Leary, M.D, and the Department had a neurophysiologist Ph.D., Dr. George Bishop, his wife, a research biochemist, who later worked with Professor Edwin F. Gildea, M.D., who replaced Dr. John Whitehorn, M.D. after he was invited to become Chairman of the Department of Psychiatry at Johns Hopkins University Medical School. Moreover, the Department had a Division of Psychology headed by Dr. Carlyle Jacobsen, Ph.D., a renowned physiological psychologist, who did the first frontal ablation experiments in subhuman animals and recorded their behavior thereafter.

The research with Dr. Felix Deutsch, M.D., (an Austrian-born medical internist who had become a psychoanalyst and was the husband of Dr. Helena Deutsch, M.D. a famous psychoanalyst too) involved looking at the blood vessels in the fingers of patients with cbronically cold hands that become worse with emotional stress (Raynaud's disease) in which he and Dr. Nadel sometimes found distorted small blood vessels, especially in the fingernail beds of these patients. Coupled with very detailed studies of the psychodynamics of these patients, photoplysmographic studies of arterial blood flow in the fingers of these patients, photos of their pathological fingernail blood vessels, and electroencephalographic studies, these men helped focus my attention--as a young medical student--on the interactions of psyche and soma. Dr. Deutsch was a fascinating gentleman. He was a piano virtuoso and used to invite symphony musicians to his apartment to play with him at the Chase Hotel complex where he lived.

With this engaging ongoing research fellowship, which was presumably a very part-time enterprise while I was going to Washington University Medical School to become a medical doctor, I can recall my learning human anatomy under the teaching of Dr. Terry (a co-author of a textbook on anatomy; he was an expert on skeletal structure) and Dr. Mildred Trotter. I remember the robust, muscular negro male cadaver to which I was assigned with a fellow male medical student. He was a graduate of Harvard University, always carried around with him a book of literature from which he frequently read. It turned out that he was going to medical school, he told me, because his parents wanted him to do so. Before the academic year was over, he convinced himself and his parents he did not want to be a physician, and, of course, he did not complete dissection of his half of the cadaver, and he dropped out of medical school. I still have the Sobotta Anatomy Atlases with most of the anatomical diagrams in color (in three volumes), which I bought second-hand, and they are possibly collector items now. Human anatomy was a complex matter of memorization, especially when it came to remembering the names of all the blood vessels, cranial nerves, sections of the brain, names of the small bones in the wrist and ankle, body musculature; and the nomenclature was all influenced bv Latin derivatives.

I learned Histology, from Dr. Cowdry and his team, and Pharmacology under the aegis of Dr. Carl Cori . Ph.D. and his wife, Dr. Gerti Cori, Ph.D. (both of whom became Nobel Prize awardees for the "Cori cycle," which describes biochemically how glucose serves as a source of energy in its metabolic cycle). And also there was Dr. Frances Graham, Ph. D., outstanding Professor of Pharmacology and the wife of Dr. Evarts Graham, M.D., Chairman of the Department of Surgery, who did the first removals of the lung (usually for cancer) and who contributed to the finding that smoking contributes to the pathogenesis of cancer, not only in the lungs but elsewhere.

And do I remember Dr. James Erlanger, Ph.D., Chairman of the Department of Neurophysiology, another Nobel Prize winner for his pioneer studies of nerves and their electrophysiological action potentials? Yes, a great lecturer and professor!

Those were noteworthy days and months and years. I was inspired by these teachers. Momentarily, my mind flashes back to some of the marvelous professors I had at Washington University as an undergraduate student, and I hear and visualize some of them who shaped my memories that are enlightened again by the current molecular biological discoveries and advances being made in genetics. I hear and see Professor Viktor Hamburgher telling us—in a special course in Experimental Embryology—what parts of the frog egg were destined to become body parts and, for example, if a barely perceptible cut was made with a glass rod (that we were taught to make ourselves) at a certain place on the egg, the embryo would develop two hearts instead of one. The scientific writings spoke about "organizers" that told the tissues what to do and in what shape to form. Today these "organizers" are identified as molecular biochemical substances, different ones for different functions and processes (identified as part of "transformation" (from DNA to RNA) and "translation" (from RNA to certain proteins) that have specific jobs to do. And Viktor Hamburgher and his colleagues did map out for us the precursor cells that were embryonic stem cells that became more and more specialized and were capable of transforming into different kinds of cells and body tissues and could replace body cells that died or had been damaged in one way or another.

Medical school was one mentally engrossing experience after another, from the basic sciences to the clinical sciences. And in many departments both basic sciences and clinical sciences were being carried out in a mutually enlightening fashion.

Residency Training and Meeting Helen Clarissa Reller

Because I wanted to be trained to become a neuropsychiatrist. I applied to Washington University, Barnes and McMillan Hospitals, to obtain training in Internal Medicine (an internship in Internal Medicine was required before beginning training in the specialty of Neuropsychiatry). My grades in medical school were good (I was elected to Alpha Omega Alpha, the Medical School scholastic honor society.) and after serving a ninth period in Internal Medicine (under the Chairmanship of Professor Barry Wood, M.D.), I began my residency in Neuropsychiatry (under the Chairmanship of Professor John C. Whitehorn, M.D., followed by the Chairmanship of Professor Edwin F. Gildea, M.D. I realize that I have already made some comments about these fine Professors, and other notable members of the Neuropsychiatry Department at Washington University, St. Louis in that era.)

Incidentally, before accepting the Neuropsychiatric residency, without applying I was invited to become a member of the Surgical residency program at Washington University. But I declined the offer, for I was firmly fixed on the idea of becoming a Neuropsychiatrist. Moreover, these years were war years. The United States of America had become involved in World War II, after the Pearl Harbor attack on some of our battleships by the Japanese, and internships and residency training in medicine were shortened from 12 months to 9 months. During the last year of medical school, we were all militarized, put in military uniforms (ASTP, which I think stood for Army Student Training Program) on a part-time basis. We were even paid a small amount of money monthly (which eased my financial shortcomings, and which was quite welcome.)

The medical internship and neuropsychiatric residency were exciting learning experiences. I could describe the learning experiences I had with different professors, but that would be lengthy and laborious—for both me and any reader—and so I will try to touch on some high spots.

One high spot was the eagerness to teach and the competitiveness to teach of two of my Instructors, Dr. George Saslow, M.D. and Dr. Daniel Badal, M.D. both graduates of the Harvard Medical School Psychiatric residency program. Both were warm and friendly men, both were married and sociable, and both enjoyed teaching. Both had had nine months of psychoanalysis with Dr. Hans Sachs, an innovation that the Harvard Program had introduced, for psychoanalysis was in its prime in ths U.S.A. The idea of self-study and self-analysis was encouraged by the educators of these two men and they fostered similar points of view in their students as well as striving to obtain the very best medical specialty education as possible—again for themselves and their students. They, too, fostered our doing scientific research and writing. Their examples and tutelage fell on fertile ground I believe, and I momentarily reflect on their personal influence on me. Daniel Badal had some neurosurgical training, and George Saslow had had some graduate education in Physiology.

There were other faculty members in Psychiatry who had influenced me: Sam Warson, A.B. Jones, Irwin Levy, Hyman Fingert, to name a few. Sam Warson supervised me on some of my cases. He was a good supervisor. But on one case in which I noted that the woman patient had a bilateral facial paralysis and I thought she had a neurological disorder, he insisted that she had a conversion hysteria. It turned out that she did, indeed, have a neurological disorder (myasthenia gravis), and she did not have a conversion hysteria. Years later, when I saw Sam Warson again while we were both attending the Institute for Psychoanalysis in Chicago, Illinois, and he was in training analysis with Dr. Emmy Sylvester, he recalled the problem we had had with the differential diagnosis on this case. Dr. A.B. Jones had a large inpatient service, many of whom were from the rural Ozarks, and he characteristically used direct psychoanalytically tuned interpretive comments on his chronic alcoholic inpatients ("Are you afraid you're a fruit?") or his inpatients with astasia-abasia and unable to get out of bed ("Are you afraid you're going to hit somebody?"). I found many of these comments embarrassing and invalid, but he was a clever neurologist and during the Grand Rounds with Neurology, Psychiatry, and Neurosurgery, he often distinguished himself as an astute diagnostician. Irwin Levy was a neurologist, and he invited me to witness his private practice at his office a couple times. He was a sharp clinician, With a fair number of outpatients with multiple sclerosis, and he emphasized that these patients were subject to remissions and exacerbations in the course of this disease. (It was not known at that time that multiple sclerosis is an auto-immune disorder in which the antibody system regards the myelin sheaths of the person's nerves as a foreign body and attacks them.)

During a busy schedule for all of us "house-officers," the hospital had a get-together and refreshments for all the doctors. At that event, I saw a very attractive blond-reddish haired woman whom I had previously noted from time to time. I introduced myself to her. Her name was Helen Reller, and I learned that she was an advanced Dermatology resident, who had also done her medical internship at Washington University Medical School. In fact, she had graduated from the Medical School a year ahead of me. I recall explaining to her later that I did not directly go to the University after graduating from high school. We immediately recognized a mutual attraction, and I was bold enough to ask her for a date. That date led to an engagement—after I met her parents and younger brother and only sibling (who was an engineering student at Washington University)—and a marriage (on August 24, 1944) at Centenary Methodist Church in downtown St. Louis.

Helen and I rented a little "efficiency" apartment at 4514 McPherson Avenue—a single room (with an in-a-door bed that we would pull down at bedtime), a tiny kitchenette, and dinette. Our residency continued, Helen rotating in Dermatology at Barnard Free Skin and Cancer Hospital, and I rotating at Barnes and McMillan Hospitals and going periodically to a St. Louis City Hospital for inpatients with tuberculosis. In September, 1946 I had to go on active military duty with the United States Public Health Service (with the rank of Assistant Surgeon—$1^1/_2$ stripes—to the United States Public Health Service (USPHS) Hospital in Fort Worth, Texas. It was a 2000 bed hospital on 10,000 acres, and it was being used by the Navy, Marine Corps, and Merchant Seaman Corps, as well as for voluntary and involuntary addiction patients (for this hospital was one of two USPHS operated Narcotic hospitals; the other one was in Lexington, Kentucky). Helen and I had to separate for she had to remain at Washington University and complete her Dermatology residency and fellowship, for she was not in the military service and had to complete full year residencies; whereas, we physicians in residency training were mandated to shorten our residencies to nine month periods so that we could be useful to our nation and our soldiers during World War II.

I had many memorable experiences as a military doctor during the next two years. In fact in 2004, I published a book on the subject entitled *World War II. Neuropsychiatric Casualties. Out of Sight, Out of Mind,* the publisher being Nova Science Publishers, Incorporated in New York. The book has sold fairly well so far. What has especially pleased me is that a Professor Jimmy Mitchell, Director of Alumni and a Professor of Mathematical Statistics, at Oxford University, London, England ordered 200 copies of this book, which Nova Science sold him at a discount ($15.00 each), and he will have to pay large shipping charges to receive the books. His plan, he tells me, is to have an "agent" of his who is involved with some of the real estate he owns in Georgia bring them to London. In any event, I am somewhat puzzled why Professor Jimmy Mitchell wanted so many copies of this book, but I expect to learn the answer to that question in the future.

I am not in the mood at this time to relate any details of my book on World War II, though it is liberally sprinkled with autobiographical comments, for while writing the book I judged that the reader deserved to know something about the personality and life of the author to help the reader understand any perspectives and biases that this single historian reporting on 1500 neuropsychiatric casualties he diagnosed and treated during his two-year tour of duty (1946-1948) at the USPHS Hospital in Fort Worth, Texas.

In Fort Worth, since I was not a high enough ranking officer in the USPHS, who were assigned good houses on the reservation, I had to find a place to live. I do not remember the details about how I found them, but the Parker family (probably recommended by the administrative staff at the USPHS Hospital) had an apartment over their garage, and that is where I lived for a while during Helen's stay in St. Louis to complete her Dermatology Fellowship. The Parkers were a congenial couple with a child; the mother was a school teacher. After Helen completed her Fellowship, she moved to Fort Worth, and we found a comfortable house to rent on Lipscomb Avenue: I think the exact address was 2814 Lipscomb, but that can be checked some time. The house was excellent; it had two bedrooms, a kitchen, a bathroom, a living room with a fireplace, and a small dining room. And it had a large backyard with some fruit trees. Helen got a position at a Fort Worth Cancer Center.

Helen and I decided to have a child. She got pregnant, and we were excited. Knowing all about the biology of embryology and the development of the fetus, and living in a place where we did not know any obstetricians, we learned that Dr. Jules Vieux, M.D., who had been one of our Ob-Gyn Professors at Washington University, had moved to Dallas, Texas, and he practiced and delivered babies at Florence Nightingale Hospital in Dallas. We contacted him, and he agreed to be Helen's obstetrician. It was quite a learning experience for me to be the father of a developing baby. To enhance my skills as a father, I adopted a cat—a male cat, yellowish-orange and white. I decided to see whether I could have the patience and skill to train this cat—we named him "Toddy"—to do tricks. I did succeed in teaching him to jump over a stick on command and to roll over on verbal and hand gesture commands. I cannot omit this little detail, and I even took some motion pictures of Toddy doing his tricks. I was so proud of this cat (and myself I guess).

Helen's pregnancy went well. Our firstborn child, Guy Henry Gottschalk, was born September 12, 1947, delivered by our friend Dr. Jule Vieux at Florence Nightingale Hospital in Dallas after a harrowing drive for me from Fort Worth to Dallas (some 30+ miles of rather rough road in those days), while Helen was having regular labor pains, and I was thinking (and worrying) that I might have to deliver the newborn. I did get to see him get born—Wow, what a tear-evoking experience to see your child coming out from the mother into this world, and hear him cry, which is good! I made it a point to see all my other children (three girls) get born—for Helen's sake and my own psychobiological state.

Before I forget the dates, and skipping ahead on this autobiography temporarily, let me record the dates of birth of my three daughters: Claire Anne Gottschalk (May 16, 1949); Louise Helen Gottschalk (March 25, 1954), and Susan Elizabeth Gottschalk (July 19, 1955).

To return to historical review, living in Fort Worth, now dwelling on Lipscomb Avenue (I have pictures of the house, one notable one of myself in my USPHS uniform standing before the front porch; how young I looked!), Helen and I had many marvelous experiences there. Helen was a outstanding cook (cuisinère). I was a boy scout cook (not very good), but I had an observant eye on those fruit trees in our backyard. They produced plums, many of them, and I decided to make some plum brandy. I studied some books, followed the directions, and made a lot of plum brandy, bottled it, and stored it under our house that had no basement. It was warm that summer, very hot, and what do you think happened? The bottles of my plum brandy all blew up. I had made root beer in St. Louis (which I even sold on the street), my brother Jules made wine, brother Edmond made some home brew (beer), and many years later (living in California) I made some very good home brew. But my plum brandy, which tasted good before it was allowed to ferment, was an amusing and explosive failure.

[At this point, I am inserting an event that chronologically does not belong here, but it occurred at this time in my historical narrative and the event has distracted me from my ordinary day-to-day life experiences, and I feel I need temporarily to make note of the matter to enable me to continue to allow my memories to come forth comfortably and smoothly.]

The Passing away of Max Jules Gottschalk

My brother Max Jules Gottschalk, as I said before, was born December 14, 1909, and he died July 26, 2005. Why insert his passing away at this point in this document? My working on this recall of memories was interrupted by the death of "my big brother" yesterday. He passed away while living, for almost three years, with his long-time companion and caretaker Robert Jackson (an ex-student in industrial design of my brother's at Pima Community College in Tuscon, Arizona) in Oxnard, California, Ventura County. Jules was a very famous industrial designer, written up in Who's Who in American Art, and the creative designer of many things—from toasters to modern furniture, automobile dashboards, to helicopters that can be flown by one person standing up on a platform over a hole in the middle of it and a propeller below it, high fidelity amplifiers with elegant record players, and so forth. For a number of years he lived in New York City and worked for Teague—a firm of industrial designers. He told me several times that the downside of his employment by a company was that with his making of successful designs he always worked himself out of a job with the company.

The passing of my brother Jules is having and will have a telling effect on me—he was my only remaining brother; but more about that later. Max Jules, during and soon after the death of his last wife—Cecile Cornsweet—told me that he wanted to donate his body to science, as Cecile did. After her death, he often shared with me that his grief over her death was difficult to bear and, finally, he joined a group of mourners who had lost a dear one, and he met with this group frequently to try to resolve his grief. He later told me that this group therapy helped him, and that his marriage to Cecile (Who was a widow, and had gone to Tucson, Arizona because her husband had painful degenerative arthritis and the warm weather in Tucson eased his pain and discomfort). Was the best of his many marriages. He was married to Josephine Pipkin, a beautiful and gifted concert pianist, not once but three times. And the third time was followed by a final divorce. Thc couple had two children: Sandra, the older child, and Jules. The second marriage was to a woman he met in New York City, and the marriage lasted less than a year. The marriage to Cecile lasted many more years (I don't know how many.)

In any event, as Max Jules was dying in a hospital in Oxnard, California, his friend and care-taker wanted to finalize the arrangements whereby his body would be donated to science. I explored the possibility of his body being donated to the School of Medicine, at the University of California, Irvine. I made contact with Michael Godsey, Director of the Willed-Body Program [(949) 824-1719; (949) 824-6061]. A Mark Brooks, the embalmer for this Program, came over to my office at the Gottschalk Medical Plaza, and he went through the legal documents with me. It asked for his legal name, date of birth, date of death, place of birth, social security number, last name of his last spouse, name of his father, place of birth of his father, and so forth. I feel my responsibilities with regards to assisting my eldest brother to leave this Earth in the way he desired has been partly fulfilled. I plan to have some kind of Memorial in his behalf. How that will involve (and include) his daughter and son and their offspring as well as other relatives and friends and acquaintances of Max Jules (Buzzy) is yet to be determined. I personally intend to organize and write a Memorial for him. It will help me resolve the details and meaning of his life and death, and I believe it will be of use to some members of my family.

Here we go again, back to the story-line. We were living in Fort Worth, Texas. Helen and I had lots of good friends there. Among the contemporaries in the USPHS were David LeGrand and his wife Alice and Gove Hambidge and his wife Elsie. David, like me, was a graduate of Washington University School of Medicine (just nine months behind me from Medical School and neuropsychiatric residency training. Gove was a graduate of Yale Medical School, and he had had some neuropsychiatric residency training in that program. And his wife, Elsie, had a graduate degree in Psychology, I believe at Yale also.

We got along well together socially and professionally. Helen and I had a baby boy while there, Gove and Elsie had a baby boy, and David and Alice had a child somewhat later. Gove's father had a position in the Agricultural Division of the United States government and for a while he was assigned to advisory activity in India. He told us about much of his activity there, including a memorable blunder he made when advising some of the people in India who were complaining about the high level of starvation in some areas because of famine, and he advised them to tie up their cattle, who had been that were roaming in their agricultural fields and eating their grain. They countered that the cattle were sacred and they could not do so. I do not remember what David's father's occupation was, all I remember about him (whom I never met) was that David said he was taught by his parents that earning interest on loans was unethical and therefore improper. I differed from David's viewpoint at that time, but I avoided talking about the matter. I think David later changed his mind when years later he bought a house in Baltimore and raised a family and became a psychoanalyst.

We all became close friends, the LeGrands, the Hambidges, and the Gottschalks. Helen became pregnant, and she bore our son, Guy. Elsie Hambidge became pregnant and had a son. The LeGrands had their children after the Fort Worth experience we all shared.

After two years at Fort Worth, diagnosing and treating mostly neuropsychiatric casualties, we had served our required tour of duty. Dr. Robert Felix, the Director of the National Institute of Mental Health (NIMH), and Dr. Seymour Vestermark and some other administrative officers, offered me and Gove Hambidge an opportunity to be the first research neuropsychiatrists at the forthcoming NIMH. We were offered further residency training, wherever we wanted to apply, as well as psychoanalytic training (at the expense of the USPHS). We both accepted the offer. I chose to go to the Institute for Psychoanalysis in Chicago (because I thought it had a more scientific orientation than the New York Psychoanalytic Institute which was very conservative at that time). Gove chose to go to the Columbia Psychoanalytic Institute in New York City (no so conservative as the New York Psychoanalytic Institute) and there were some famous child psychoanalysts there (including Dr. David Levy), in which Gove was interested. I ended up getting child psychiatry residency experience at Michael Reese Hospital in Chicago as well as adult and child analytic training at the Institute for Psychoanalysis in Chicago. I had a traning analysis with Dr. George Mohr (as I mentioned in the beginning of this document on Memories) and some notable supervising analysts (who supervise your treatment cases—"control" cases). I had Dr. Thomas French, Dr. Margaret Gerard, Dr. Adrian Van der Veer, Dr. Emmy Sylvester, Dr. Louis B. Shapiro, even Dr. Franz Alexander, Dr. Theresa Benedek, Dr. Roy Grinker, and Dr. Jo Ann Fleming. There were others, whose names I may remember later. It was a splendid experience. I had to learn to live and survive in Chicago (with its very hot and cold, windy weather). Helen and I lived in Brainerd, a suburb of Chicago, and I commuted by train (the Chicago Rock Island), bus and street car, and sometimes by automobile (in a Chevrolet car we bought). We rented a second-floor apartment from the Giganti family in Brainerd. I will never forget trying to put skid chains on my car to drive to downtown Chicago, in the winter snow and ice. I had to use my auto when going to my psychoanalyst's house in the Hyde Park area of Chicago because it was difficult to get public transportation there. When I saw Dr. Mohr at the Institute for Psychoanalysis on 110 Michigan Avenue, I could use some form of public transportation. As I briefly reflect on it now, that was character building—contributing to perseverance, a trait I still have.

Helen and I had another child (Claire Ann) in Chicago. Helen got a fellowship at the University of Chicago, working under the aegis of a prominent dermatologist; she did some key work on acetyl choline and its role in skin function. The Chairman of the Department of Obstetrics and Gynecology delivered our new baby; I watched her being born. (I remember Helen's mother (Frieda) scolding her for getting pregnant a second time (I am sure she meant well. I came from a family of four children and uncle Louis had twelve children. And Helen's parents had two children, Helen and Charles ("Chuck"). Helen and I both wanted to have a least two children, maybe four.)

Toddy our big unaltered male cat was with us. The Giganti father complained that Toddy urinated on their porch and yard (sending messages that he had marked his existence). We tried to keep him indoors as well as we could. Since Helen and I both had positions, we had to figure out how to get baby-sitters. A nearby mailman's wife helped out occasionally. And they steered us to an Irish Catholic policeman (whose job was to serve as a guard at one of the city jails) and his family, and they served us well. Now Helen and I had two fine youngsters, and we enjoyed ourselves with them, going to the Lake and swimming, going to the great Lincoln Park Zoo, the Museum of Science and Industry, the Field Museum, some art museums, and driving around the city and countryside.

Then in 1951, it came time for us to move to Washington, D.C. and the National Institute of Mental Health. Its planned location was Bethesda, Maryland. We headed for that area and eventually found a house being built on Persimmon Tree Road in Potomac Village, Maryland, off the junction of Bradley and River Roads. That was our first house, not well built; because when it rained or was otherwise moist, the floorboards kept popping up. I would have to get under the crawl space and with Helen's help up on the floor level, I would drill holes through subflooring and floor and pull the floor boards down. I remember the County required, as well as the lender who had a loan on our property, that there had be a walk to the house and I built one out of big flat stones we bought. Helen and I worked and built and painted (we added a room in the garage) and even added a toilet and sink in the area of that new room. It was amateurish but suitable.

The children were marvelous. Helen and I loved those days. Even Harry Reller, Helen's father, came there to visit us and helped us work on our one-half acre backyard. I built a big tree-house for the kids (just as we used to do for ourselves at the Mutrux's ten acres).

At NIMH, I was the first neuropsychiatrist there, for Gove Hambidge came along later. I decided to continue to work on research I had started and published on while at Michael Reese Hospital in Chicago: psychological trigger mechanisms in epileptic seizures. A mentor of mine, Dr. David McK. Rioch, had a position as Director of Research at Walter Reed Army Hospital in Silver Spring, Maryland, and he was also associated with Chestnut Lodge, a private neuropsychiatric hospital in Rockville, Maryland. He made it possible for me to see psychiatric patients who had epileptic seizures—some of whom had had the stressful task while on military duty of defusing bombs that, for one reason or another, had not exploded. I would have these inpatients talk about these stressful experiences or any other ones while I recorded their electroencephalograms (EEGs), and everything they said. Examining the transcripts of these verbal recordings and at the same time their EEGs, I searched for any possible and recurring connections between what the patients were saying and any EEG abnormalities that occurred simultaneously or immediately following verbal evidence of anxiety or hostility. Eventually that led to my making a career specialty of trying to specify the form and content of speech and verbal behavior that provides criteria for measuring the magnitude of emotions and many neuropsychiatric dimensions, Dr. Rioch encouraged and facilitated my research. After Gove Hambidge arrived at NIMH, I persuaded him to focus also on verbal behavior during the associative process. At the time, we looked at words (rather than on grammatical clauses, which I later focused on), and published a paper on our findings, in which we noted that different interviewers elicit different verbal behavior from the same speaker (and later that some interviewers elicit more anxiety from the same individual than others.) [Louis A Gottschalk and Gove Hambidge, Jr. Verbal behavior analysis; a systematic approach to quantifying psychologic processes. Journal of Projective Techniques. 19:387-409, 1955]

Helen and I were very happy with our children and our life in Bethesda, Maryland and Potomac Village, and Guy started school in Potomac Village. But my salary from the USPHS service was limited by a ruling from the newly formed National Institutes of Health that a physician could not--even on his or her own time—do private practice and receive compensation from that practice. I was seeing some psychoanalytic patients and obtaining some supervision from some of the local famous psychoanalysts (Dr. Edith Weigert, Dr. Frieda Fromm Reichman) and paying for supervision, but not being allowed to charge fees from the patients.

After being at NIMH for two years, I began to receive invitations from several Medical Schools and Universities to accept an academic position. There were invitations from the Department of Psychiatry, Downstate New York Medical School, from Washington University Medical School in St. Louis, from the Medical School in Chapel Hill, North Carolina, and from the University of Cincinnati School of Medicine. Helen and I decided to go to the University of Cincinnati because they offered a "geographic full-time appointment," both to me and to Helen from the Department of Dermatology, and the Cincinnati group was affiliated with the Chicago Institute for Psychoanalysis. Dr. Maurice Levine, Chairman of the University of Cincinnati Departmant of Psychiatry had had his training analysis from Dr. Franz Alexander, who became the Director of the Chicago Institute for Psychoanalysis.

So I went to Cincinnati with the position of Research Professor of Psychiatry. And Helen got an academic position as Associate Professor of Dermatology. We moved to Cincinnati in 1953 (having been in the Washington, D.C. area from 1951 to 1953), and we lived there from 1953 to July 1967 and had two more children, a daughter Louise Helen (born March 25, 1954) and a daughter Susan Elizabeth (born July 19, 1955). In July 1967, I was invited to become the Founding Chairman of the Department of Psychiatry and Human Behavior, College of Medicine, University of California in Irvine, California—where I am today. But before I get to that exciting period of my life, I should elaborate on our family life in Cincinnati, a city and time period we all dearly loved. We bought a large home built in 1929 (from the owner, who told us it cost $75,000.00 to build) 3828 Clifton Avenue, adjacent to a little side street, Rural Lane. (Physicians eventually occupied all the homes on Rural Lane, 4 psychiatrists, a pediatrician, a surgeon, a general practitioner—except for the house directly across from us on Rural Lane). Our house was magnificent, constructed by German craftsmen, three stories above ground with beautiful oak floors, a full basement, 22 closets, five bedrooms, a huge living room, a dining room, and a large study on the first floor. The price tag (a lot of money in those days) was $37,500.00, so we had to borrow some money. (We sold this fine house in 1967 for $45,000, and we had to pay $55,000.00 for the house we bought at 4607 Perham Road in Corona del Mar, California, which was on rental land; we eventually bought the land for $31,500.00.)

The years (1953 to 1967) in Cincinnati were quite eventful. Academically, I was a success. I obtained many NIH grants, did much research and teaching, and collaborated with a number of people including Goldine C. Gleser, Ph.D. a research psychologist from Washington University, St., Louis, whose doctorate was in mathematical statistics and psychology. I benefited from her creativity and statistical expertise, and, in addition to journal articles, we published a ground-breaking book (Louis A. Gottschalk and Goldine C. Gleser. *The Measurement of Psychological States from the Content Analysis of Verbal Behavior.* Berkeley, Los Angeles: University of California Press, 1969.) In addition, working with another collaborator, Carolyn Winget, we published another significant book (Louis A. Gottschalk, Carolyn N. Winget, Goldine C,. Gleser. *Manual of Instructions for Using the Gottschalk-Gleser Content Analysis Scales: Anxiety, Hostility, and Social Alienation-Personal Disorganization.* Berkeley, Los Angeles: University of California Press, 1969.)

During the Cincinnati years, Helen and I were both prolific, family-wise, academically, professionally, and socially. In between bearing two daughters, Louise and Susan, Helen taught Dermatology, did clinical research, published actively, and did some dermatological practice. I taught, did basic and clinical research, got many research grants, became a supervising and training psychoanalyst with the Institute for Psychoanalysis in Chicago. The latter position required my periodically traveling to Chicago (by train or by plane) for what was named "geographic training analysis programs" in those days. (The Institute for Psychoanalysis in Chicago fostered several budding psychoanalytic institutes in various cities—Cincinnati, St. Louis, Cleveland, and Rochester and, hence, the term "geographic" was somehow invented and applied to ongoing psychoanalytic training programs in those cities.). I often went to New York City or other cities in various roles—to serve on NIH research study sections (which studied and reviewed training and research grant applications for NIH), to attend professional scientific meetings, to participate in furthering psychoanalytic education in conjunction with the American Psychoanalytic Association, to serve on Committees of the American Psychiatric Association, American Psychosomatic Society, American Psychoanalytic Association, the Association for Research and Mental Disease (ARNMD), and so forth. Because I became the key person to do so, I organized the beginnings of the Cincinnati Psychoanalytic Institute—which required some legal documentation involving the city of Cincinnati as well as some reviews and appraisals from the American Psychoanalytic Association. (I wonder whether that legal and professional documentation still exists.)

While living in Cincinnati, Helen and I got the idea of looking around and buying a farm somewhere. It was my idea. The Mutrux family had a ten-acre farm where they reared their 12 children, and we Gottschalks spent a fair amount of time there. Our parents were close to one another and that could be a factor. In addition, my mother one summer sent us for two weeks to Cottage Farm, an arrangement whereby farming families would have children stay with their family and see and learn what farm life was like. Charlie, Edmond, and I were left with a farm family that had cows, a horses and a mule, and cultivated their land, growing corn and lots of vegetables. The farmer's children were friendly and sociable. We were taught to milk cows, and feed livestock, and they let me ride a mule (all by myself) to the nearby town and post-office. The mule was a lot of animal for me to manage. It would walk slowly and sometimes would want to turn and go home; the boys told us to show the mule who was in command, and it worked. Another factor could have been my experiences at a Boy Scout camp Where I sometimes was a camp counselor. I also had been a camp counselor at a private camp (Camp Nebagamon in northern Minnesota, near Duluth. Where I had been responsible for the youngest boys ranging in age from 7 to 9), all Jewish children. The camp was beautiful and we could arrange to go on trips with a horse and wagon, cook out and sleep out. The rural country-side was fascinating. Helen and I examined several farms, discussing the pros and cons of each one. We finally settled on buying a 180 acre farm in rural Indiana, in Ripley County. It had 100 acres of forest, and a large stream (Laughery Creek) flowing on one side of it. It included two large barns, one for livestock, and the other for farm equipment and machinery. These farms were obviously built by hand, with large and long beams fastened together with wooden pegs. The farmhouse, a sizable log cabin, was covered on the outside with flat boards, by the person who sold the farm to us. The house had a side porch. The seller said he bought the farm at a County sale, because the previous owners could not pay their taxes. He was happy about the sale to us (for $10,500.00), and we were happy about our purchase. I borrowed some money to pay for the farm, and after several years I was able to pay off the loan. Helen and I and our children loved going to the farm. We made friends with our neighbors including (George Hartwell and his wife and daughter—with whom we became close friends. He helped us farm the property, plant corn, soy beans, tomatoes, even raspberries). And then there was the Lauber family, who also farmed their land; the father worked for the Ripley County Road Department. We learned that farm life was hard if you tried to make a living out of it. But if you had another source of income—as Helen and I did—in a sense, farming was an avocation. The winters were cold and uncomfortable, and the roads were difficult to traverse. I bought a pre-owned Ford tractor, a wagon, a large cutter that had to be connected to the tractor. We would invite our friends (often the Wingets, sometimes the MacLeods and Ordways) and many of our children's friends to come out to our farm and have picnics and ride in the flat bed wagon pulled by our tractors over the Ripley County back roads. During the summer season we had feasts of our own fresh sweet corn, tomatoes, cucumbers, and barbecued chicken. George Hartwell got us to raise hogs, and he would look after them when we were back in Cincinnati. George was partially deaf, from a childhood infection, but he could read lips. He was a very intelligent man; who wrote and recited a lot of poetry. His uncle had been a political figure in Ohio (Hartwell County). I bought a hearing aid for him, but he did not like it because it was too noisy, and he figured he could do just as well without it. Helen and I had unforgettable experiences on our Indiana farm. We have pictures of some of it, I am glad to say. For a while, I had my brother Edmond live on the farm. He was very handy in many ways. He installed an indoor toiled, shower, kitchen sink, and built a new cistern (fed water from the roof top of our farmhouse). One can never forget the luxury of an indoor toilet, but we soon learned that an indoor toilet needs water to operate successfully, and that was very difficult to accomplish, especially in winter when all of the water in the pipes (copper) Edmond and I installed froze and so became blocked and unusable.

George Hartwell became so close to our family that he asked whether he could come to Guy's wedding to Ann Schieble in the San Francisco area at a Catholic Church Seminary. He rode all the way from Ripley County, Indiana on his Indian motorcycle to attend the wedding ceremony. Incidentally, his daughter was accepted on a scholarship to the University of North Carolina in Chapel Hill. Of course, I wonder what has happened to her. I believe she was interested in forestry and wanted to be a forest-ranger as a teenager.

There are many priceless memories associated with our Indiana farm. With the help of the United States Department of Agriculture, I learned that an American citizen could purchase at a very low price thousands of little trees and plant them on bare gound . We did so, ordering and planting fir trees, pine trees, and walnut trees. Planting them by hand was tedious, but we did so for a small number. We got someone to plant many of them using a tractor. Growing trees is a long-term project. I do remember visiting our farm periodically and even once after we had sold it and moved to California. The pine trees, once little Christmas trees, had grown to about a hundred feet in height.

George Hartwell persuaded us to raise hogs. He built pens for them and arranged their water supply. I recall holding a male piglet while he castrated it to make it grow larger. I recall having a cement truck bring a load of cement so that Guy and I could have it pour a load so we could build a large concrete front porch. I planned and helped to build, with the aid of a large earth moving machine, two dams to collect rainwater that could be stored in two large ponds, and from those ponds we drew water to supply the hogs and other livestock we acquired (a palamino gelding and a mule for George to use). I bought a gasoline engine pump to pump the water into tanks. I bought a gasoline powered engine to run a generator to supply us with electric power. Helen and I were Sears Roebuck customers, and we acquired some equipment and the ability to run our farm. All these farm activities were sandwiched in with our activities in Cincinnati with our medical school and medical practice roles. We entertained frequently in our large residence. In our front room we had a huge fireplace, and George Hartwell would bring us cords of firewood to use for the fall and winter seasons. I insisted that my children take music lessons, and I purchased a baby grand walnut Baldwin piano. (I brought that same piano to California; we loved it and played it frequently. Only my daughter, Susan, became proficient at the piano. Louise played the violin for a while.) I took piano lessons myself, and I got fairly good at the piano. Helen had piano skills, and we worked on playing some duets, especially Mozart duets. I then got into playing the classical guitar, influenced some by my first cousin, Paul Mutrux, who had become a guitar virtuoso as well as achieving many other skills. (Many members of the Mutrux family had musical aptitude and skills.) I bought a fine Martin classical guitar, took guitar lessons, and I learned to play a number of pieces and some of the Carcassi exercises. (Somewhere, I have records of a Russian expert playing many of the Carcassi exercises.)

My father visited us in Cincinnati several times. He painted some landscapes in Cincinnati (one of which I still have), and he painted some still lifes (flower pictures), and he painted a picture of people skating on the lake in Forest Park, St. Louis, in front of the St. Louis Art Museum on Art Hill. I have that very painting in my study in my home at Corona del Mar, California.

Dean Warren Bostick, M.D., of the College of Medicine, University of California Irvine came to Cincinnati, and he persuaded me to accept the Founding chairmanship of the Department of Psychiatry and Human Behavior, of the fledging University of California at Irvine, in 1967. He promised that Helen would have an academic position in the Department of Dermatology, which she did, indeed, obtain. A new chapter in our lives evolved with our move to California.

CALIFORNIA AND OUR LIVES THERE

Helen and I had been to California a number of times, specifically to San Francisco and to Los Angeles. There were professional meetings in California, for example, the American Psychiatric Association, the American Psychoanalytic Association, the American Psychosomatic Society, that we attended. I recall that at one of these professional meetings, a friend, Dr. Fred Kapp and I decided to take a break briefly from a meeting in Los Angeles of the American Psychoanalytic Association and visit Disneyland—in Orange County, California—and that was the first time I had ever been there. I never imagined that I would, many years later, return to Orange County and live there many years, if not the rest of my life. And there was that marvelous experience with David and Alice LeGrand, when we were on our way driving down the Oregon and California coast in 1944 on our way to Fort Worth, Texas—David and I scheduled to report for active duty at the USPHS Hospital. I will never forget that experience—especially, when we went through San Francisco. Helen, brave woman, resolved to swim in the Pacific Ocean, and sure enough, as we drove near a beach in San Francisco, Helen put on her bathing suit and went into the Pacific Ocean. She said it was cold, but she loved it. No one else was swimming at the time from that beach. Helen did.

The University of California at Irvine, under leadership Warren Bostick's Deanship of the College of Medicine, arranged to move all of our belongings to Irvine, California. The moving expenses must have been large. Everything we wanted to move to California, the State of California moved for the University of California, including our baby grand walnut piano, two large wagon wheels from a farm planter, a large hand drilling tool used in barn and house building to drill holes through large wood beams, a fortyish pound iron bell that I had mounted on a 15 foot high post to tell our family members and friends that it was a meeting or dinner time at our farm. Even after 1967, I still have some of these items, except for the Baldwin walnut grand piano, which I recently sold, for no one used it any more, because some of the strings were broken by our living close to the Pacific Ocean. Claire sold the piano for me, finding a piano teacher, who checked the identification number of the piano, played it, told her he wanted it and would fix the piano himself. He offered her $3000.00 for it, got herself a commission of $600.00, and in about a week that beautiful piano was gone from our home at 4607 Perham Road. But that happened in September 2005. Let us go back to our experiences at Irvine, California.

Helen and I searched for a house. We found a suitable one, within our means at that time, in a subdivision named Cameo Shores in Corona del Mar, California. It was located three streets from the Pacific Ocean, in our vicinity each street had been built on a street overlooking the street in front of it so that the ocean view was not impaired. One could see Catalina Island (25 miles across the sea) and even San Clemente Island (100 miles away) on a clear day. The house was a flat-roofed oblong building with sliding glass windows on the ocean-side and permanent wall-sized glass windows in the living and diningroom and, a bedroom on the opposite side. The house needed remodeling and we did that. Over several years we added a study with a closet and bathroom, an enclosed breezeway, an attractive redwood ocean-side front deck. Oh yes, we upgraded the kitchen and the dining area with bookshelves and compartments with glass covers for our collection of Mexican, pre-Columbian, and Indian vases and artifacts.

We built a concrete block wall on the right side of our house separating our yard from the house on the right of us (from the Perham Road viewpoint). On the Perham Road side we erected a high (about 8 foot) concrete block wall with tall doors on either side of a three-car garage. The house cost us $55,000.00, and it was on rental land. We bought the land later for $31,500.00. All these money details amounted to a lot of money for us, but we gradually paid off this indebtedness. I mention these details also because the real estate values and prices have soared remarkably in Southern California since our coming there.

Susan and Louise started school at Lincoln School. They liked it. They told Helen that some of the other girls at school made fun of their beautiful dresses and clothes, many of which Helen made for them. I reflect now that kids mostly girls often do that—that is, they want all other kids in their age range to be clothed and, otherwise, look similarly. Helen was, indeed, a remarkable woman. Her sewing machines were also shipped from Cincinnati to California, and I can readily recall going with her to various nearby stores with her that sold all kinds of clothing materials, threads, and dress patterns. She continued to make or redesign the clothing of our children, the three daughters and also our son. She had a large collection of cookbooks (over 20) that she consulted often. And this same woman was a Phi Beta Kappa member, an Alpha Omega Alpha (AOA) medical honorary society member, an outstanding dermatologist, and a Clinical University Professor! What a fortunate man I was to have found and married her!

Helen did get a University of California position as Dean Bostick had promised. She was in the Department of Dermatology, headed at that time by Professor Gerald Weinstein, M.D. who later became Dean of the College of Medicine, Dr. Weinstein's wife was a clinical psychologist. Her son went to UCI College of Medicine, got a medical degree and also, a doctorate in Biochemistry under the aegis of Dr. Dennis Cunningham, now an Associate Dean. This son is now a faculty member and neurologist at the University of Washington in Seattle. Dr. Weinstein's wife died of two cancers, sad to say. Later Gerald Weinstein asked me whether one ever gets over the death of a loved spouse, and I said that could take a while. He still sees patients at UCI, and he has told me that he remarried; he married the wife of a dermatologist who had died, and that she is a psychologist. I gather he is happy or happier now. But like me, I am happy but very much miss my Helen, who died May 28, 1993 suddenly of a ruptured pulmonary aortic an eurysm that had not been detected even though she had had a pre-fatal pulmonary x-ray which did not reveal the pulmonary aneurysm. But let us return to the marvelous experiences that Helen and I had together from 1967 to 1993 in California. (I took a short break to have a bite of lunch at this point, eating a donut my daughter Claire brought with her and her dog—Brooke—for a walk to look at the ocean and its waves. In the brief interim the thought occurred to me—in visual form—of figures on the walls of caves of humans and animals drawn by ancient cave dwellers; those distant ancestors were recording things, events, and life forms long, long before I did. What I am doing in recording these memories is a genetic manifestation of the way we are made. The Egyptian pyramids with their drawings and figures, the Inca pyramids and their drawings, the gods that humans invent and worship, the figures or statues symbolizing and representing ideas and forms of life—these all represent a process that is motivating me to continue to record what I am naming my memories.)

Well, Helen and I had our hands full in an exciting way. We had together these four children we had conceived, and we had the responsibility of earning a livelihood for them as well as ourselves, and we had the job of obtaining a shelter for all of us—now in our house in California.

Our daughter Claire had been initially left behind in Cincinnati. She had insisted on marrying a boy she met in Cincinnati. When she told Helen she loved this boy and wanted to marry him, Helen asked me whether we should put Claire in a mental hospital? All I could think of to reply was what was happening to Claire was "love" but that you could not hospitalize someone for falling in love. I did not say "it's all chemical" though at one level of thinking that is true and so is writing and thinking, breathing, looking, and sleeping and being awake. Claire after a while in Cincinnati got pregnant, had a baby girl, Tracy, and separated and divorced her husband, who got involved with drug abuse. Claire joined us with Tracy. Tracy went to school at a Montessori school, while Claire went to nursing school—I think it was Saddleback Junior College-and eventually got training in nursing of patients with chronic diseases. Tracy, for a while, went to Corona del Mar High School, graduated and later went to Saddleback Junior College. Around that time she fell in love with a young man who got involved with alcohol and drugs. She lived with him in a duplex I owned in San Clemente. Somehow during these tough financial times, she did well academically at Saddleback Junior College, and she was accepted for admission to the University of California at Berkeley, California. Tracy and her boyfriend moved to Oakland, California. Tracy liked Berkeley, did well there academically, majored in History and aspired to do graduate studies in History at City University College of New York. By this time, a break-up of her relationship with her boyfriend had occurred, and she went to New York, taking with her a dog, whom she still has, who helped sustain her during her stay in New York. The graduate work in History did not last long, and she decided to return to California and pursue education to become a high school teacher. She got her teaching credentials at San Francisco State University, and for many years she has been teaching high school in Santa Clara County. At her invitation I have visited the high school where she teaches, and there she has gained a very respectable reputation as high school teacher and administrator. And the dog whom she loves, who went with her to New York, is still with her. (Her mother—Claire—with whom I went on a walk with her dog, Brooke, told me today—April 2, 2006—that Tracy a few weeks ago had to have her dog put to sleep because of paralysis. The dog was 17 years of age.).

Tracy has had some stressful experiences during her life in California, but the purpose here is not to write about her life. That is a project for her to develop and work on some time in the future. She has a success story, which is well beyond my scope.

My daughter Susan, a gifted artist and musician, went to the University of California at Santa Barbara. Helen and I used to ride there to visit her and that beautiful country-side. Parenthetically, let me say we even poked around and looked at some residences for sale in that vicinity and even some rural land in San Luis Obispo available for farming and raising cattle. I remember the agent took me to a cattle auction which fascinated me. But reality reared its head, and I looked at the enterprise and scenery and backed off getting further involved.

Susan did very well academically at the University of California, Santa Barbara. There she encountered Marston Smith, and they fell in love and got married. Marston was one of the offspring of a father (Mortimer, I believe) who was a physicist, a graduate of Brown University, who worked for IBM and had worked on plans for a space station. His wife (Betty) was also a Brown graduate, a philosopher, a Greek scholar, and a Jungian, and later a Jungian psychoanalyst. Their son Marston (I think there were at least two daughters), like his father (who was a music lover—he was an expert on the clavichord) was a fine cello player. He decided he had to study cello further with a member of the Beaux Arts Trio in New York. Susan and Marsden decided to transfer to Stony Brook University on Long Island. They both got admitted to Stonybrook, and Susan continued her University undergraduate work there with honors, Marsden bought an expensive cello, and became a pupil of the virtuoso cello player in the Beaux Arts trio. Susan became pregnant, bore a son who got named Hampton (the name of a village near Stony Brook) and after Susan's graduation, the couple returned to California to live for a while with the Smith family on their farmland in upper Malibu. Later, Susan, Marston, and baby Hampton moved to 424 Fernleaf, in a duplex Helen and I owned, and Claire lived in the adjoining duplex apartment (424 1/2 Fernleaf in Corona del Mar, California) with Ray Weaver whom she had married. Tracy lived with her mother while she went to Corona del Mar High School and occasionally when she went to Saddleback Junior College, before she went to Oakland, California to attend the University of California, Berkeley. Ray was a business man, made a fairly good living, was a sailboat devotee, and had many friends. He developed multiple sclerosis, could not tolerate the crippling effects of multiple sclerosis had on his physical prowess (especially being unable to play golf or manage the physical prowess required for racing sailboats), and he hung himself in their garage. Poor Claire said she had to cut him down. Now she lives fairly comfortably with a man she has known for 13 years, Robert (Bobby) Moore, a construction worker.

Susan and Marston, for reasons I do not well understand, got a divorce after some marriage counseling, which was unsuccessful. Susan said that Marston was self-centered and tended to be preoccupied with himself and his musical ventures. Susan went to work in a business in which she arranged and photographed weddings and their locations. She also was very prolific in experimenting with art and invented a type of art in which in glass-covered boxes were used to present various picturesque displays of objects, several of which I have in my possession. She also did some novel things with photographic film in which she pushed around the photographic gel on film used in immediate photography (designed by the Kodak company). She was able to make a livelihood in these artistic enterprises, and she was even able to obtain a Masters of Business Administration (MBA) from Pepperdine University (August 8, 1981). How she accomplished these feats while nurturing and rearing her boy, Hampton, is a wonder. She became romantically involved with a young man in the Marine corps stationed, I think, at El Toro. They planned a marriage, and at first their plan was to live at Susan's duplex apartment in Corona del Mar, which Helen and I owned. I believe her fiancé had some reservations about having a step-child (Hampton)—as many prospective and actual spouses do with regards to a step-child. In any event, he insisted, for some reasons that I never learned about, to live in Lancaster, California, It may have had something to do with where he might have been able to get employment; whereas, Susan wanted to remain in the vicinity of Newport Beach and Laguna Beach, where she had most of her clientele and friends. Claire now tells me that Susie had chronic low back pain, for which she had a surgical procedure, that bothered her and that may have depressed her. But Claire herself suffered a spinal cord injury and surgery from an auto accident that certainly influences her point of view about Sue's state of mind. After writing a book of poems, which are somewhat on the melancholy side, and leaving a number of farewell notes to her fiancé and family, she committed suicide by shooting herself in her head. How tragic to all of us! It was little Hampton, who, unable to get into their duplex home because the door was locked, climbed into her bedroom window and discovered his mother's body. What a traumatic effect that had on my little grandson Hampton! He was a grandson whom I had to father (joyously) after his own father, Marston, was separated from my dear Susan. Marston remarried a woman named Betsy who looked very much like Susan. They had two children together, who live with Betsy and their grandmother, Betty Smith. Recenly, Marston separated and divorced Betsy. I believe another woman is involved with Marston, but I avoid talking about this with Hampton. Hampton has been attending the University of California at Berkeley and getting high honors. He is expected to graduate with a major in environmental science. [a degree similar to one received by Erin Gottschalk, my eldest granddaughter has, Who got her degree from the University California at Davis, and has an excellent job in this field.] Hampton at this time has gone to Tahiti for 10 weeks to attend a University of California sponsored course in his major—Environmental Science. He tells me he plans to do a research project on this island to which the French artist, Paul Gaugain, has attracted our attention.

I communicated with Hampton via his email address (Hampton@uclink4.berkeley.edu) while he was in Tahiti. He did research on a small form of marine life and wrote an excellent paper about its eating patterns and prey; I have a copy of the paper. While there, he and his classmates and their professor went to an island prized and owned by Marlon Brando. Hampton and his classmates surfed and scuba-dived about the small island, and he commented that the sea was warm and underwater sights and flora were magnificent. He returned to UC Berkeley for a short time, and then he went to Budapest to take a five-month history class, his final class at UC Berkeley, I understood, to obtain his BS degree.

Sara Gottschalk, the youngest daughter of Guy and Ann, graduated from Sage High School, a private school in Irvine, California, and she is now attending Orange Coast Junior College. Maybe I will follow up on telling about her. But I should first tell more about the lives and professional careers of Helen and myself in California.

The Department of Psychiatry and Human Behavior, College of Medicine, University of California at Irvine, in 1967, needed accredited adult and child psychiatry residency programs. It also needed a location where neuropsychiatric outpatients and inpatients could be seen, diagnosed, and treated. Also needed was an Emergency Reviewing and Admitting Unit. Those goals were initiated and accomplished at the University of California Medical Center in Orange, California. A large structure (building #53) was earmarked for those tasks. It was a three-story building with a large basement. I believe, somewhere, I have already written a document reporting the history of the Department—at the request of the University of California administration—and I will see whether I can locate it. Here it is.

Notes on the Beginnings of the Department of Psychiatry and Human Behavior, College of Medicine, University of California; Irvine, California

To make understandable the beginnings—and to a large extent the current structure—of the Department of Psychiatry and Human Behavior at the University of California, Irvine, I believe it would be helpful to describe briefly my own education and training before coming to UC Irvine as Founding Chairman in July, 1967.

I received a Bachelor of Arts in July 1940 from Washington University, St. Louis, Missouri, with a triple-major: English, Biology, and Experimental Psychology. Then I went to Washington University School of Medicine in St. Louis, and during my medical school education I had a Josiah Macy Foundation Fellowship in Psychosomatic Medicine doing research in the Department of Neuropsychiatry, which at that time was headed by Professor John Whitehorn, M.D., who later became Chairman of Psychiatry at Johns Hopkins School of Medicine. My research in the Neuropsychiatry Department was under the direction of three famous people: Professor Felix Deutsch, M.D., a prominent Viennese psychoanalyst and physiatrist; Professor Carlyle Jacobsen, Ph.D., a neuropsychologist (who did, among other things, the first frontal lobe ablation studies in animals at Yale); and Professor David McK. Rioch, M.D., (a neurologist and neuroanatomist, known for his seminal research on the extrapyramidal system). Dr. Whitehorn, who had initially been a biochemist before becoming a neuropsychiatrist, was replaced as Chairman at his departure from Washington University School of Medicine, by Professor Edwin Gildea, M.D., also initially a biochemist, from Yale, who had become a neuropsychiatrist. That Neuropsychiatry Department was, clearly, a combination of psychiatrists, psychoanalysts, neurologists, neuropsychologists, neurophysiologists, and biochemists. That conception of what faculty members belong in a department of Neuropsychiatry was imprinted on my brain, and I still carry it with me. My residency training in this Department was accredited in both psychiatry and neurology.

After graduation from medical school, during World War II, I served as a neuropsychiatrist at the United States Public Health Service (USPHS) Hospital) in Fort Worth, Texas, a 2000 bed hospital for acutely psychotic Naval and Marine Corps personnel and for narcotic addicts. (Before World War it had been a Federal Narcotic Hospital located on 10,000 acres.). During my two years there, I was allowed to take a three-month Fellowship in Electroencephalography at Washington University School of Medicine under the guidance of Professor George Bishop, Ph.D. (a famous neurophysiologist) and Professor James O'Leary, M.D. (Head of the Neurology Division of Neuropsychiatry), to help me direct the Electroencephalography Laboratory at :the USPHS Hospital in Fort Worth, Texas. From this Hospital I went to Michael Reese Hospital, Chicago and the Institute for Psychoanalysis in Chicago to obtain certified training in Child Psychiatry and Adult and Child Psychoanalysis. I, also, directed the EEG Laboratory at the Institute for Psychosomatic and Psychiatric Research and Training at Michael Reese Hospital.

From 1951 to 1953, I was the first research neuropsychiatrist at the National Institute of Mental Health, Bethesda, Maryland.

From 1953 to 1967, I was Research Professor of Psychiatry, College of Medicine, University of Cincinnati. In Cincinnati, I was also a Training and Supervising Psychoanalyst with the Institute for Psychoanalysis in Chicago, which in those days was a prestigious, research-oriented psychoanalytic institute, which appealed to me, under the direction of Dr. Franz Alexander, M.D. and Dr. Thomas French, M.D.

Warren Bostick, M.D., Dean of the College of Medicine, University of California, Irvine, personally came to Cincinnati, Ohio to recruit me. He persuaded me to become Founding Chairman of the Department of Psychiatry, promising me not only a Hospital and Clinic (actually, he promised a Neuropsychiatric Institute similar to the ones at UCLA and UCSF, funded I learned not by the Regents of the University of California but by the Mental Health Division of the State of California), but also Biochemistry and Neurophysiology Laboratories (including animal research facilities) and a generous budget for clinical and basic research personnel and clinical faculty. I convinced him of my own conviction that Neuropsychiatry was not only a clinical medical science, but also a basic medical science! I arrived in July 1967 to assume my administrative responsibilities and build a department based on my concepts and experiences in Neuropsychiatry. I had been offered other Chairmanships, but these were at universities (for example, New York University, the State University of New York in Brooklyn, the University of North Carolina at Chapel Hill, the University of Maryland) that were already existent and had been headed by other chairpersons. Here was an opportunity to organize and develop a department from its beginning. I did not have to worry about trying to remedy the problems left by other chairpersons. I had an opportunity to be creative at the great research University of California, in a state that was financially supportive to education and its universities. In what directions should I go and use the resources that were available to me?

On reflection, I realized that I could not predict where the biggest advances were likely to be made in Neuropsychiatry. I knew I wanted there to be a strong commitment to research, some of which my budget could support, at least at the beginning. I knew that there were available large amounts of federal, state, and county moneys to support research for enterprising and qualified faculty neuroscientists. I knew we had to obtain approved residency training programs, in Adult and Child Psychiatry. I knew we had to organize an educational program for our medical students. I knew that UCI was taking over (buying) the

Orange County Medical Center and that our initial patient source was going to be the Mental Health Hospital portion of the Orange County Medical Center. It seemed not only possible but appropriate to go in many directions to reach the goals of a strong research department in clinical and basic behavioral sciences, an outstanding educational program for medical students and residents-in-training, and diverse neuropsychiatric patient responsibilities.

I find it enjoyable to review what happened 30 years ago during my 12 years of Chairmanship of our Department of Psychiatry and Human Behavior, a department name already given to it when I arrived. The experience was challenging and fun, and the outcome was quite successful. There is space here only to cover the high points.

Challenging Situations

(1) In taking over the Mental Health program at the Orange County Medical Center, we inherited a Psychiatric Emergency Admitting Unit that saw 800-1000 patients per month, including acute alcoholics, drug-abuse patients, patients with all neuropsychiatric disorders, and many neurological and medical disorders. The Unit was great for teaching, but heavy with respect to responsibility, including lawyers looking for reasons to sue.

(2) The California Lanterman-Petris-Short bill provided large amounts of moneys to California Counties for broad mental health care. We sought and obtained a large amount of these funds and supported many clinical faculty members and mental health educational programs in Orange County. The challenging events were: (a) Research was looked upon with suspicion, the argument usually being "we know everything; let us put the money into treatment and not waste funds." (b) The Orange County Board of Supervisors came up with the notion that there were no mental health problems among Orange County children! So funds did not need to be allocated for absent problems. (We got the Orange County League of Women Voters to do a study on this issue, and they reported that Orange County had as many mental health problems among children as other Counties in California. So, we eventually got our share of financial support in this clinical area.)

(3) There were over 300 full-time employees at our Mental Health Hospital, servicing the needs of patients on a 24-hour/day basis. Personnel problems did occur and had to be attended to.

(4) Our successes in taking over various residency training programs as well as clinical programs (Veterans Administration Hospital, Long Beach; Metropolitan State Hospital, Norwalk; Student Mental Health Services at California State University, Fullerton and at Orange Coast Junior College and University of California at Irvine, Orange County Community Mental Health Programs in Costa Mesa, Fullerton, and Orange, and so forth) provided us large amounts of funds to use for research and training. But these responsibilities required administrative and clinical care over more than a one-hundred and fifty mile area.

Fun Situations—Including Recruiting, Growth, and Achievements

(1) We obtained basic science laboratories both at UCIMC (Biochemistry laboratory and a Neurophysiology, EEG, and Computer Laboratory).

(2) The Beckman Instrument Company gave us $250,000.00 worth of laboratory equipment (which amounted to a lot of equipment in our new departmental laboratories).

(3) When the building Medical Sciences II was completed, the Department of Psychiatry not only got many laboratories there, but an equipment budget from the University of California, Irvine, budget.

(4) Our Department was the most successful Department of the College of Medicine with respects to obtaining extramural research and training grants.

(5) Our Department obtained funds for the first extramurally supported Research Center on the UCI campus, namely, an Alcoholism Research Center (Funded by the National Institute of Alcohol and Alcohol Abuse (NIAAA), Scientific Director—Louis A. Gottschalk and Scientific Co-Director--Sujata Tewari) made up of faculty members from the Departments of Psychiatry, Psychobiology, Molecular Biology, and Biochemistry. It focused on the effects of alcohol on the nervous system.

(6) Our Department obtained a second extramurally supported Research Center (Funded by the National Institute on Drug Abuse (NIDA), Director—Louis A. Gottschalk) focused on the causes of psychoactive drug-related deaths and the development of a system of uniformly recording the relevant information on these cases across the U.S.A.

(7) Several faculty members received Research Career Development Awards from NIMH, NIAAA, or NIDA.

(8) We obtained approval from the American Psychiatric Association and the American Boards of Psychiatry and Neurology, Inc. for adult and child psychiatric residency programs.

(9) We were so successful in obtaining residency applicants that we were given the opportunity to take over the residency programs at Metropolitan State Hospital, Norwalk, CA. and at the Veterans Administration Hospital, Long Beach, CA. We specified that funds from Metropolitan State Hospital for residency training should include a budget for research and research facilities at Metropolitan State Hospital, including Biochemistry and a Psychology Laboratories. The same requirements were exacted of the Veterans Administration Hospital, Long Beach. Department faculty members located at these places were encouraged and allowed to apply, respectively, for research funds from the State of California, Mental Health Division and the Veterans Administration Hospital.

(10) The Department took over the training of our residents at Capistrano-by-the-Sea Hospital, specializing in drug-abuse problems, alcoholism, eating-disorder problems, and general adult and child psychiatric disorders. The Department also developed a Free Drug Abuse Clinic for children in Laguna Beach, CA.

(11) Recruiting good faculty was successful. For example: Arnold Mandell was recruited from UCLA; he later left our Department to become Chair of Psychiatry at UCSD. Mansell Pattison was recruited from the University of Washington, Seattle; he later left our Department to become Chair of Psychiatry at the Medical College of

Georgia. Ernest P. Noble was recruited from Stanford; during his tenure at UCI he served for a few years as Director, NIAAA and, then, after returning to UCI, he accepted a name-Chair in Alcohol Research in the Department of Psychiatry at UCLA. John Kramer served several years during his tenure in our Department in Washington, D.C. in the Drug-Abuse Advisory Unit during the Nixon Administration. Gordon Globus was recruited from NIMH, and he directed our program at Capistrano-by-the Sea Hospital. Three faculty members (Roger Walsh, Mansell Pattison, and Louis Gottschalk) obtained joint-appointments in the Schools of Social Science and Social Ecology, and they participated in the doctorate programs of these divisions, that is, they were responsible for several doctoral students. Other psychiatry faculty members had joint appointments in other Departments (for example, John Kramer in Pharmacology, Ernest Noble in Psychobiology, Sujata Tewari in Molecular Biology and Biochemistry). A few faculty members were Training and Supervising Psychoanalysts for the two Los Angeles Psychoanalytic Institutes: Justin Call and, years later, Richard Fox and Mark Markowitz (two ex-residents), for the Los Angeles Psychoanalytic Institute. Gilbert Morrison and Louis Gottschalk and, later Richard Gelker and Jeff Seitelman (two ex-residents) for the Southern California Psychoanalytic Institute.

(12) Many resident graduates have achieved academic success. For example, David Shore went to NIMH, and he now has a high-level staff position there. John Schwartz became editor and publisher of the highly successful and popular Psychiatric Times, which many people thought was superior and more informative than the monthly American Psychiatric Association's American Psychiatric Association News. Ken Globus became a member of the Psychiatry faculty at UC Davis. Other ex-residents are now on Psychiatry faculties elsewhere.

(13) At its peak in residency numbers, there were well over 60 psychiatric residents in training under our Department's auspices.

(14) The Department had quite sizeable training grants, especially from NIMH, but also from NIDA and NIAAA, the Veterans Administration, and the State of California, Mental Health Division. Most of these training grants were for residents. Some were for medical students.. Some were for medical specialists (for example, pediatricians, family and general practitioners, even one for anesthesiologists) who wanted to obtain specialty training in Neuropsychiatry! (I believe such matters have changed today.)

(15) Stanley van den Noort was Chair of Neurology at that time. He wanted Psychiatry to combine with his Department and become one department. At that time, mainly because of wide differences in funding in favor of Psychiatry, I did not see that this arrangement would be wise. (I do not think Dr. Van den Noort liked being turned down on his request; I may have made a mistake at that time.)

(16) Most faculty members had individual and sizable research and/or training grant funding. Research, education, and clinical service activities of the Department were flourishing in the middle and later 1970's. Several faculty were serving on the American Psychiatry and Neurology Board examination Committee. Several were on the Editorial Board(s) of refereed journals. Several faculty members won national recognition awards for their innovative research. Several faculty were on

regular Extramural Research Review Committees or Study Sections of the National Institutes of Health.

(17) Relationships with the community were good. More than 200 volunteer clinical faculty members became involved in the teaching activities of the Department. The Orange County Psychiatric Society was organized and developed under the leadership of the Department, and many faculty have served on the Council and/or as officers of this Society. Some faculty members had top clinical leadership or administrative roles in the Orange County Mental Health Department's clinical activities.

(18) Several refereed journals had their editorship located in our Department: for example, The American Journal of Drug and Alcohol Abuse and Psychoanalytic Education. Later, Psychiatry Research (under Monte Buchsbaum) had its editorship in our Department. Many faculty members were on the Editorial Board of journals, such as, Archives of General Psychiatry, Psychiatry, American Journal of Psychotherapy, Methods and Findings in Experimental and Clinical Pharmacology, Biological Psychiatry, Psychosomatic Medicine. Many faculty did ad hoc evaluations for such journals as Science, New England Journal of Medicine, American Journal of Psychiatry, Nature, and so forth.

(19) Overall, the Department of Psychiatry and Human Behavior from 1967 through 1978 was, in the opinion of the Founding Dean, Warren Bostick, of the College of Medicine, one of the strongest Departments in the College of Medicine. (I have just learned that Warren Bostick, M.D. the Founding Dean of the College of Medicine at UC Irvine, died 3/18/06 in Northern California according to an email note from our current medical school Dean Thomas Cesario, M.D.). It may seem I am reporting this lightly, but I was quite sad to learn about it, for he was an important and very significant person—as well as a friend—in my life.

To return to the narrative of my autobiographical memories, after being relieved of the administrative responsibilities of being the Chairman of the Department of Psychiatry and Human Behavior at UC Irvine, I continued as Professor Emeritus, and I continued to do research, publish papers, book chapters, and books, and I continued to see adult and child patients.

My dear wife died, unexpectedly on 5/28/93, after phoning me from our home at 4607 Perham Road, Corona del Mar, when I was at UCI and telling me “Louie, I think I’m having a heart attack!” I rushed home and learned that she had been taken to Hoag Hospital in Newport Beach. I rushed to the Emergency Room there, and I learned that she had died. An autopsy showed a ruptured pulmonary thoracic aorta—a finding that was completely unexpected, for she had recently had a pulmonary X-ray read by the Chief of Pulmonary Medicine, and it was negative for any pathological disorder of that sort.

Helen and I had briefly and casually discussed what we should do if either one of us predeceased the other. She said she loved the location and Pacific Ocean so much where we lived that she wanted to be cremated and have her ashes distributed in the Pacific Ocean. We had a funeral ceremony on a special boat, and I scattered her ashes in the Pacific Ocean. (I have not thought about that melancholy detail lately, but that is what I want done with my remains and in that form rejoin Helen.) It took me almost a year to carry out her wishes, for I kept her remains at my home, and then I finally did what she requested. Of course, I miss her very much, but I am comforted by my rich memories of all the marvelous times we had together, the trips we made, the homes we lived in, the children we had, and the unforgettable experiences we all had together. I live alone in our home at 4607 Perham Road, Corona del Mar, California, and I find myself talking to her and expressing my endearing nicknames to her when completely awake and, from time to time, when I am going to sleep or awakening from sleep. I ask myself what would people say if the they heard me talking that way, and I answer they would understand and, if not, that would not make any difference to me. Doing so I re-experience the enduring love involved in our marriage. The calender details of our marriage (Marriage date August 24, 1944 at the Centenary Methodist Church in St. Louis, Missouri, and her passing away May 28, 1993.). We had known each other intimately over fifty years. I have no desire to remarry. But I notice I am still attracted to women of all kinds--children and adults. I had a wonderful mother, a loving wife, three beautiful daughters, some fine female first cousins (three of them--Mutrux). Moreover, that should be no surprise. I am a male.

When Helen passed away, I reflected how I could make a permanent memory to her and myself and our marital union, maybe in some philanthropic way? Both of us, were financially unable to afford going to Washington University undergraduate and medical school, but were helped by scholarships and loans and by achieving academic recognition in the forms of Phi Beta Kappa and Alpha Omega Alpha (the medical school scholastic honorary society) I reasoned that helping some other students obtain a professional education would be the right way to go and appropriate. Through hard work and successful stock and bond investments as well as real estate investment, I decided, with the legal help of a lawyer friend (Berneice Anglea) to donate some funds to the University of California, College of Medicine, at Irvine—a one and a half million dollar donation (specifically, the Louis and Helen Gottschalk, Charitable Remainder Unitrust)-- to be made available to whatever or whomever the contemporary Dean of the College of Medicine at UC Irvine decided—after my life is terminated. In recognition of this philanthropic contribution, the administration at UCI Irvine decided to name the medical outpatient clinic on the UCI campus the GOTTSCHALK MEDICAL PLAZA. Helen was a well recognized and outstanding Clinical Professor of Dermatology, and I was a Professor Emeritus of Psychiatry and Human Behavior and recipient of the University of California Irvine Medal (for my neuroscientic and neuropsychiatric achievements and publications), and this was the other underlying reason for the UCI administration naming the first medical outpatient clinic on the UCI campus the GOTTSCHALK MEDICAL PLAZA. The Chancellor at UCI Irvine at that time was Dr. Karen Wilkening, Ph.D. This building is an attractive glass-topped building (I should find out who the architect was and when the building was completed.) where I have an office and where I see my outpatients regularly. I am certain Helen would approve of and be proud of the GOTTSCHALK MEDICAL PLAZA.

About this time (1994), I established the Gottschalk Family Partnership, a legal entity of which I was the General Partner and my offspring (Guy Henry, Claire Ann, Louise Helen, and Susan Elizabeth) and their children be Limited Partners so that the federal taxes on my estate be significantly reduced at my demise. The overall estimated value of the California real estate was about $2,000,000.00 in 1994. The funds donated to UCI came from the sale of stocks and bonds, which funds were transferred to the Northern Trust Bank, which are invested by this bank in a special fund that will be turned over to UCI when I pass away. Under ordinary circumstances earnings from the real estate (currently, the home where I live—4607 Perham Road—which is now owned by the Gottschalk Family Partnership and for which I pay monthly rent to the Partnership, two mini-storages [one in Beaumont, California—Xenia Stor-All--and one in a suburb of San Diego—Troy Street Mini-storage], one condominium, and an eight-acre Organic Avocado Ranch in southern San Diego County [the Valley Center area] with one legally buildable lot on it.). It was Berneice Anglea who recommended and legally arranged the Gottschalk Family Partnership in order to reduce the federal inheritance taxes when I die, for my children and grandchildren will inherit a large percentage of this Partnership.

I should mention here that while I was awarded a Fellowship at the Rockefeller Study and Conference Center for six weeks in Bellagio, Italy in 1985, and Helen joined me and sincerely loved the place and location, I met many distinguished scholars—also enjoying a Fellowship like mine. Among the scholars was a Nigerian gentleman and academician, who invited me to visit Nigeria and told me, among other matters, of oil wealth that had been discovered in Nigeria. He suggested I might want to be an investor in Nigerian oil wells, and invited me to form a company, Export LLC, which could make money by being an agent for such companies as John Deere and Caterpillar Tractor Company and any other bulldozer companies whose equipment could be used for road-building and other enterprises in Nigeria and were difficult for Nigeria to obtain from the U.S.A. To generate funds for my family, I formed this company. My Nigerian friend, whose name I forgot, contacted me and eventually I visited his colleagues who traveled to meet me in the Ivory Coast rather than Nigeria (because a dangerous battle was going on in between warring factions in Nigeria), signed some contracts, and because of the amounts of money involved to be wired to Export LLC (millions of USA dollars), they persuaded me to pay a premium payment to the National Insurance Company of Nigeria (NICON) to guarantee and protect the payments to me. To make a long story short, over a ten-year period, I spent over $1,000,000.00, dealing by fax and telephone with various Nigerians (my original Nigerian friend had died). My son, Guy, and my daughter Claire—after studiously examining the Gottschalk Family Partnership annual tax reports---brought a conservatorship lawsuit against me as the general partnership, questioning my capacity to function as the general partner and seeking for Guy and his wife, Ann, to assume the functions of the general partner. Guy's lawyer brought two lawsuits, one in terms of a breach of "fiduciary duty" and the other seeking to function as the general partner. The initial hearings on the two lawsuits denied the contentions of the two lawsuits. The media (the Los Angeles Times, initially) published the news about the lawsuits—with such headings as "Acclaimed Psychiatrist and UCI Professor scammed by Nigerians according to a lawsuit brought by his son, Guy, also a doctor." I was tempted to omit this matter from this autobiography, but the newspaper publicity, was repeated throughout the USA and spread to a number of foreign countries (Germany, France, Japan, et cetera). So I decided this was an historical detail, and there was no use in trying to cover up the matter. I had many calls from friends and acquaintances all over the USA about the situation, who read their local news media, and they had the general attitude that I was more to be pitied than scorned and how sorry they were that I lost money on such an investment. Many tried to comfort me by saying that other people have lost money on investments at one time or another too. And since some of the newspaper articles reported my net worth was in the realm of multimillions of dollars, not much more was said. Now I believe a court settlement has been made, requiring me to have a family memher (Guy, Claire, Louise) co-sign the checks I write for the Gottschalk Family Partnership, which is quite acceptable to me. In any event, little did I expect those marvelous weeks Helen and I spent together in Bellagio, Italy at the Rockefeller Study and Conference Center would eventuate in such a Gottschalk family legal squabble and alienation.

During the years after Helen passed away, I busied myself by involving myself in medical research, writing, publishing, and seeing and diagnosing and treating medical patients. I have been heavily involved in these activities. As a faculty member at UCI, it is an obligation to keep a curriculum vitae (CV), which lists my various academic and clinical medical appointments, my journal publications, my book chapters, and the books I have published or edited, the presentations or lectures I have given at various universities or professional meetings. I enjoy these activities. There are well over 200 journal articles, over 100 book chapters, and over 35 books. In a way, my CV summarizes my professional and academic memories. I think of including my CV here, but I soon reject including a 75+ page document of this sort into this autobiographical narrative because that is too narcissistic at this point, though there is healthy narcissism and self-love. But this is not the best place and time for including such a document, and who would want to read it?

I have had many grants and awards, federal, state, county, and from foundations and companies. I do not want to list these but rather I want to relate the research work that has interested and engaged me over the past 35 years. That is, the content analysis of natural language and verbal texts, covered by the publication with Goldine C. Gleser, by the University of California Press in 1969, *The Measurement of Psychological States Through the Content Analysis of Verbal Behavior*. That work, plus my teaming up with Robert J. Bechtel, Ph.D., a computer scientist, about 20 years ago, has led me to write an article entitled *Computerized Psychodynamic Psychotherapy* which summarizes the fascinating studies with which I have been involved over the past two to three decades.

The aim is the development of computer software that will be capable of performing like a neuropsychiatric diagnostician and psychotherapist, will remember what the subject/patient has typed into the computer in response to queries and prompts introduced by the computer over many occasions, will recall and record all the neurobiological scores the individual has made over all these occasions, and can illustrate the ups-and-downs of the individual over some 30 different neurobiological dimensions, and which of these scores are one to three standard deviations over norms we have found for the scores on these dimensions. It will indicate what the computer therapist has said in reaction and response to the subject/patient responses, and the details of the dialogue between these two participants. I am looking for a break-through with this software and the methodology it manages, for no one has yet accomplished such a feat.

Computerized Psychodynamic Psychotherapy

Introduction

The computerization of psychotherapy involving a health provider and a patient is a challenge that was introduced and pioneered in 1966 by the publication of Eliza (Weizenbaum, 1966). A computer program capable of providing psychotherapy to the diversity of personalities likely to test and use such a program, a program at the same time prepared to adapt to the wide variety of mental conflicts and disorders for which an individual might seek treatment, is far from being accomplished at this time.

Not all mental or physical disorders are capable of being changed or remedied. Which are responsive to treatment and which are not are issues and matters that are worth determining.

Therapy aims to modify and relieve distress, discomfort, and pain in addition to arriving at a diagnostic evaluation and classification. Psychotherapy attempts to achieve such a goal through empathic listening by a well-trained and licensed specialist (for example, psychiatrist, neurologist, psychologist, psychiatric social worker) who uses various verbal techniques, taught by different theoretically based schools, which need not be reviewed here. Other therapeutic procedures directed at mental disorders include neuropsychopharmacology, electroshock and other cerebral electromedical procedures, and cerebral neurosurgical approaches. Moreover, various religiously based methods, guided meditation, worship of statues, religious confession and absolution, the influence of rocks, special stones, jewelry, and photographs and pictures are claimed to have therapeutic value.

Methods and Procedures

The computerized diagnostic and therapeutic program described here is not capable of substituting for the expertise of a medical doctor (or other professional person) who is qualified to know what to do with an individual who has a potentially dangerous medical or neuropsychiatric illness. When the possibility of a serious medical disorder (such as cancer, cardiovascular problem, cerebral vascular stroke, congestive heart failure, infection) or serious mental disorder (potentially suicidal, homicidal, gravely disabled mentally or intoxicated from alcohol or other drug abuse) is discovered, the subject should be immediately advised to consult a physician and/or appropriate professional specialist.

Under ordinary circumstances, a clinician has several options in obtaining objective and valid clinical evaluations. For example, precision and accuracy may be avoided and impressionistic reactions may be relied on. Some clinicians feel they are able to do competent clinical work with an impressionistic approach. Another clinician can spend considerable time and care in the diagnostic and therapeutic evaluation of patients with the goal of assessing accurately and precisely the magnitude of diverse medical and psychopathological processes within and across patients at different times.

Another diagnostic approach is to use various observer psychiatric rating scales, such as, the Brief Psychiatric Rating Scale, the Hamilton Anxiety or Depression Rating scales or various self-report measures, such as, various adjective checklists. Although such measures are widely used in many clinical research projects, their use carries with them a false sense of security since quite often no inter-rater reliability tests are done with the rating scales, the assumption being that anybody can follow the instructions for rating and no measurement errors are likely to occur. With rating scales, however, raters vary widely on how much of the range of ratings they use with the same subjects. Some raters characteristically select the lower range of the ratings, whereas others habitually choose the higher range of the ratings. With self-report measures, the assumption is the self-raters are all, indeed, in good and equivalent contact with themselves and are not likely to be falsifying, consciously or unconsciously, their self-evaluations, though it is true that the self-rating comes directly from the individual being evaluated.

These kinds of measurement errors in observer rating scales and self-report scales, usually disregarded by researchers and clinicians, are minimized in the measurement method of content analysis of verbal behavior. The individuals being rated are usually not aware what speech content or form is being analyzed, and they have difficulty covering up, even if they have some notions about such matters. Furthermore, the unstructured approach customarily used to elicit speech avoids the questionnaire or cross-examining method, and allows the subject to elaborate and use free-will to the extent desired by the self on choice of topics on which to verbalize. Emotions, self-reflections, doubts, and defensive maneuvers are recorded, and these all contribute to the content analysis scores eventually recorded and calculated.

In previous research, we have made some progress along this pathway that will be summarized here. Initially, there was the creation, development, and validation of the measurement of the magnitude of psychobiological states and traits from the content analysis of verbal behavior by human scoring (Gottschalk and Gleser, 1969; Gottschalk, Winget, Gleser, 1969). In these and subsequent reports (Gottschalk, 1979; Gottschalk, Lolas, Viney, 1986; Koch and Schofer, 1986; Gottschalk, 1995, 1999, 2000), the objective measurement from the content analysis of verbal behavior was validated for the content analysis scales for the following categories:

Anxiety Scale. The type of anxiety that this scale measures is what is sometimes labeled free anxiety in contrast to bound anxiety, which manifests itself in psychological mechanisms of conversion and hypochondriacal symptoms. Some aspects of this anxiety scale are registered by other phenomena, such as, displacements (verbalizing about others or the environment manifesting fearful behavior or activities) or denials (asserting without being asked that one was not scared or anxious). The Anxiety Scale is classified into six subtypes: death, mutilation, separation, guilt, shame, and diffuse or nonspecific anxiety. Fear of death is assessed by content items dealing directly with death and destruction. Mutilation anxiety is manifested by allusions to fear of injury. Separation anxiety refers to fear of separation, abandonment, or loss. Guilt anxiety is defined through verbal references to adverse self-criticism, abuse, self-condemnation, moral self-disapproval. Shame anxiety is identified by expressions of self-ridicule, feelings of inadequacy, embarrassment, humiliation or exposure of personal shortcomings. Diffuse or nonspecific anxiety is identified by such references as "nervous" or "jittery" or "rattled."

Hostility Scales. The hostility scales are designed to measure three types of hostility of a transient rather than a sustained affect. Hostility scores derived from several lengthy verbal texts from an individual will provide a trait-like measure.

Hostility Directed Outward Scale measures the intensity of adversely critical, angry, aggressive, assaultive, asocial impulses and drives towards objects outside oneself.

Hostility Directed Inward Scale measures degrees of self-hate and self-criticism, and to some extent feelings of anxious depression and masochism.

Ambivalent Hostility Scale measures not only some aspects of hostility directed inward, but at the same time it measures some features of hostility directed outwards.

All three hostility scales assign higher weights to scorable verbal statements communicating hostility that, by inference, are likely to be strongly experienced by the speaker; whereas completely repressed hostility is not scored.

Social Alienation-Personal Disorganization Scale. This scale was originally designed to measure the relative degree of personal disorganization, social withdrawal or feelings of isolation of schizophrenic persons. The common denominators of the schizophrenic syndrome are considered to be disturbances in the coherence and logicalness of thinking process and deficiencies in human relationships, especially those manifesting in alienation, avoidance, and antagonism. Another principal characteristic of the concept of the schizophrenic syndrome is that it is a syndrome that is quantifiably describable, that is, there are relative degrees of severity of schizophrenia. In some schizophrenic individuals this severity can fluctuate considerably from day to day. This concept of schizophrenia, in fact, holds that these principal characteristics and features of schizophrenia—social alienation and personal disorganization—occur to mild degrees and to a varying extent in nonschizophrenic individuals, but not in such a continuous and/or extreme fashion in schizophrenia itself (Gleser, Winget, Seligman, & Rauh, 1979; Gottschalk and Gleser, 1969; Winget, Seligman, Rauh, & Gleser, 1979).

Cognitive and Intellectual Impairment Scale. The Cognitive Impairment scale is designed to measure transient and reversible changes in cognitive and intellectual impairment as well as permanent and irreversible changes, all due principally to brain dysfunction and minimally to emotional changes in the individual.

Depression Scale. The Depression scale provides dimensions that are compatible with the concept that there are a number of potentially relevant subcategories of constructs of depression that have significant statistical relationships with different underlying pathogenic processes (Gottschalk, 1966). Thus, in addition to providing a total depression score, it has a broad range of phenomenological subscales. These are: Hopelessness, Self-Accusation, Psychomotor Retardation, Somatic Concerns, Death and Mutilation Depression, Separation Depression, and Hostility Outward.

Hope Scale. The Hope Scale is designed to measure the intensity of the optimism that a favorable outcome is likely to occur, not only in one's personal earthly activities, but also in cosmic phenomena and as well as spiritual or imaginary events. A high hope score is intended to be of predictive value with respect to human survival, the preservation or enhancement of health, or the welfare or constructive achievement of the self or others (Gottschalk, 1974; Gottschalk, Bechtel, Buchman, Ray, 2004).

Human Relations Scale. The Human Relations Scale measures the relative inclination an individual has to care about and be interested in and help others. It is a scale that measures the degrees of altruism a person has.

Achievement Strivings Scale. The Achievement Strivings Scale aims to assess the achievement motivation of an individual. It notes the relative degrees of motivation one has mentally and physically and it records and measures various kinds of deterrents and blockages to such achievement-orientations.

Dependency Strivings and Frustrated Dependency Scales. These scales focus on verbal references to dependency wishes and frustrated dependency.

Health/Sickness Scale. The Health/Sickness Scale measures the relative preoccupations of a person with health and heathfulness versus sickness and ill health.

Quality of Life Scale. The Quality of Life Scale measures the relative quality of life an individual reveals based on the content analysis of what they say or write. A review of the criteria on which this scale is based is available in Gottschalk, Bechtel, Buchman, Ray (2003b). It is derived from content analysis scores from the Human Relations Scale, the Hope Scale, the Social Alienation-Personal Disorganization Scale, the Depression Scale, and the Health/Sickness Scale.

Scoring Norms

Norms (mean score and standard deviation from the mean) have been established for most, though not all, of the scales. The norms are derived from human-assigned scores. The norms have been shown to vary with age (adult/child, with a cutoff at > 18 years), gender, and (for some scales) ethnicity.

Norms for the various scales, by age and gender, are given in the table 1 below. On samples where information is not available about subject age and gender, the adult male norms are used for comparison.

Table 1. Norms for the Gottschalk-Gleser Content Analysis Scales

	Male Adult		Male Child		Female Adult		Female Child	
Scale	Mean	S.D.	Mean	S.D.	Mean	S.D.	Mean	S.D.
Anxiety Total	1.48	0.70	2.05	0.89	1.48	0.70	2.05	0.89
Death Anxiety (1)	0.30	0.51	0.55	0.45	0.18	0.34	0.63	0.42
Mutilation Anxiety (2)	0.36	0.55	0.79	0.63	0.28	0.51	0.92	0.67
Separation Anxiety (3)	0.30	0.46	1.18	0.78	0.42	0.52	1.16	0.55
Guilt Anxiety (4)	0.31	0.49	0.41	0.22	0.31	0.47	0.43	0.32
Shame Anxiety (5)	0.42	0.57	0.95	0.69	0.70	0.70	0.80	0.59
Diffuse Anxiety (6)	0.35	0.46	0.55	0.27	0.45	0.63	0.69	0.45

Table 1. (Continued)

	Male Adult		Male Child		Female Adult		Female Child	
Hostility Outward Total	0.97	0.50	1.15	0.58	0.97	0.50	1.15	0.58
Hostility Outward Overt	0.70	0.36	0.80	0.48	0.70	0.36	0.80	0.48
Hostility Outward Covert	0.67	0.46	0.86	0.48	0.67	0.46	0.86	0.48
Hostility Inward	0.60	0.35	0.74	0.54	0.60	0.35	0.74	0.54
Ambivalent Hostility	0.58	0.43	0.68	0.38	0.58	0.43	0.68	0.38
Social Alienate-Personal Disorganize	-2.89	2.70	-1.15	4.75	-2.89	2.70	-1.15	4.75
Cognitive Impairment	0.81	0.47	2.51	1.80	0.81	0.47	2.51	1.80
Hope	0.74	1.03	0.05	1.25	0.74	1.03	0.05	1.25
Depression Total	5.48	1.87	6.16	2.82	5.39	1.53	6.37	2.37
Dep - Hopelessness (I)	0.90	0.31	0.98	0.54	1.05	0.38	1.15	0.53
Dep - Self-Accusation (II)	1.03	0.58	1.11	0.86	1.41	0.76	1.25	0.75
Dep – Guilt	0.37	0.21	0.47	0.18	0.41	0.18	0.50	0.53
Dep – Shame	0.79	0.53	0.83	0.80	1.18	0.78	0.85	0.83
Dep – Hostile Inward	0.64	0.38	0.77	0.45	0.75	0.33	0.72	0.30
Dep -Psychomotor Retardation (III)	0.35	0.10	0.41	0.16	0.41	0.19	0.42	0.28
Dep – Somatic Concerns (IV)	0.34	0.10	0.54	0.32	0.46	0.17	0.51	0.33
Dep - Death/Mutilation (V)	0.93	0.65	0.88	0.78	0.57	0.40	0.86	0.79
Dep – Death	0.65	0.50	0.52	0.33	0.48	0.28	0.56	0.35
Dep - Mutilation	0.70	0.50	0.84	0.70	0.46	0.35	0.75	0.70
Dep - Separation (VI)	0.86	0.63	1.02	0.75	0.71	0.35	0.94	0.43
Dep – Hostility Outward (VII)	1.06	0.56	1.23	0.62	0.77	0.33	1.19	0.46
Dep - Hostility Out Overt	0.72	0.36	0.89	0.49	0.69	0.31	0.88	0.45
Dep - Hostility Out Covert	0.81	0.51	0.84	0.60	0.50	0.19	0.80	0.39
Health/Sickness	0.65	0.40	0.65	0.40	1.40	1.10	1.40	1.10
Health	0.43	0.34	0.43	0.34	0.94	1.09	0.96	1.09
Sickness	0.22	0.24	0.22	0.24	0.46	0.34	0.46	0.34
Human Relations	0.99	0.76	1.78	0.61	1.40	0.95	1.78	0.61
Achievement Strivings	1.11	1.17	1.11	1.17	1.11	1.17	1.11	1.17
Achievement - Support	1.84	0.99	1.84	0.99	1.84	0.99	1.84	0.99
Achievement - Deterrents	0.74	0.54	0.74	0.54	0.74	0.54	0.74	0.54
Dependency Strivings	0.54	0.42	0.54	0.42	0.54	0.42	0.54	0.42
Frustrated Dependency Strivings	0.11	0.18	0.11	0.18	0.11	0.18	0.11	0.18
Quality of Life	-1.67	3.71	-1.67	3.71	-1.67	3.71	-1.67	3.71

The content analysis approach to the measurement of psychobiological dimensions includes the strengths of both the self-report approach and the observer rating scale approach, and minimizes the weaknesses of both in terms of measurement errors. Of particular interest in the current setting is that content analysis is particularly well suited for use in dialogue systems, which typifies psychotherapy.

To address training and performance obstacles to wider use of the content analysis scales, we developed and tested software capable of reliably scoring computer-readable transcriptions of verbal (speech) samples on the Gottschalk-Gleser scales (Gottschalk and Bechtel, 1982, 1995). Computer scoring was accomplished over a number of years (Gottschalk, Hausmann, Brown, 1975; Bechtel, 1982; Gottschalk and Bechtel, 1982, 1989, 1993, 1998-2002; Gottschalk, Bechtel, Maguire, Katz, Levinson, Harrington, Nakamura, Franklin, 2002; Gottschalk, Bechtel, Maguire, Harrington, Levinson, Franklin, Caracamo, 2000; Gottschalk and Gottschalk, 2002;Gottschalk, DeFrancisco, Bechtel, 2002; Gottschalk, Lolas, Viney, 1986; Reynolds, 2001: Lavid, Grayden, Gottschalk, Bechtel, 2001; Maguire, Gottschalk, Riley, Franklin, Bechtel, Ashurst, 1999). In operation, the program (called PCAD, for Psychiatric Content Analysis and Diagnosis) assigns scores on the user-selected scales to each clause in the input sample, then, at the user's option, reports score summaries for each scored scale with comparisons to established norms for the subject's demographic group, provides an analysis of the score profile, and suggests possible diagnoses drawn from the Diagnostic and Statistical Manual of Mental Disorders, Fourth Edition (DSM-IV) (American Psychiatric Association, 1994). In addition, computerized scoring of these content analysis scales during conversational interactions was achieved (Gottschalk, Bechtel, Buchman, Ray, 2003, 2004).

A quick review of the steps the PCAD program takes in the process of measuring the relative magnitude of diverse neuropsychobiological states and traits would be helpful at this point.

The software system relies on a reasonably sized dictionary (~200,000 words) marked with associated parts of speech, and a collection of (mostly American) English idiomatic and slang expressions. Some of the words and all of the idioms have been manually identified as possible indicators of semantic content relevant to one or more of the scales. Syntactic information such as part of speech and number is extracted from the dictionary and used by a parser that outputs an analysis of the structure of each input clause.

When a word or phrase in an input is found in the dictionary as a possible marker of an item from a scale, a partial score is added to a list of scoring candidates. This list of candidates is then examined by a set of scale-dependent procedures that consider the clause structure as well as the scoring candidates to decide the validity of each potential score. For example, the speaker must be the recipient of an action or affect described in a clause for the clause to be scoreable on the Hostility Inward scale, while the speaker must not be the recipient on the Hostility Outward scale. Candidate scores approved by this process are emitted as content analysis scores applicable to the input clause, together with weighting as defined by the scale. Scores for individual clauses are aggregated to provide an overall score for the sample.

A scoring summary is prepared for each active scale. The summary gives tallies of the number of occurrences of the various tags, a word count, and a single score based on scale-specific tag weightings that is used to characterize the verbal sample on each scale. The human scorer of content analysis can distinguish semantic messages being communicated in context across several grammatical clauses; whereas, the software program analyzes the meaning conveyed by context only within each grammatical clause. Thus, computer scoring may miss some aspects of the meaning being conveyed when two or more clauses are required to discern the meaning communicated in context across several grammatical clauses (e.g., "I was very frightened by the situation. It was new to me. I don't think I could become accustomed to that.") Thus, computer scoring may miss some aspects of the meaning being conveyed when two or more clauses are required to discern the meaning. For this reason, the software system does not always precisely match scores assigned by trained human scorers. Since the tagging dictionary was developed manually, occasional errors occur. Some tagging categories require judgments that we have been unable to capture in programmatic form. For example, on the Social Alienation/Personal Disorganization (Schizophrenic) scale, a clause is to be tagged if it contains "Obviously erroneous or fallacious remarks or conclusions; illogical or bizarre statements." To accommodate these differences, the score produced by the software is adjusted to create a "human equivalent" score, with the adjustment derived from a human and computer scoring of a set of 71 samples maintained as a standard.

We have developed regression formulas enabling us to convert computer-derived content analysis scores into human-equivalent scores by scoring large numbers of verbal samples both manually using human experts in scoring and automatically using the computer program. These computer-to-human conversions provide some correction for the problem of missed scores. Since the norms we have obtained for the content analysis scale scores from adults and children are based on human expert scorers, the machine-derived scores may be compared to the human-derived norms whenever it is desirable to determine how many standard deviations from our norms any newly obtained content analysis scores may be.

Not all of the scales have conversion formulae, so not all have human equivalent scores. No conversion to human-equivalent has been established for the following scales:

- Health/Sickness
- Human Relations
- Achievement Strivings
- Dependency Strivings and Frustrated Dependency Strivings
- Quality of Life

The computer-to-human conversion factors are calculated separately for each scale and subscale. The factors are given in table 2 below.

For those scales (above) with established computer-human conversion factors, the human-equivalent score is used for testing against norms. For scales with no established conversion from computer-generated scores to human-equivalents, the computer-generated score is used directly for comparison to the mean.

Table 2. Computer-Human Conversion Factors

Scale/Subscale	Multiplier (slope)	Offset (y-intercept)
Death Anxiety	0.92	0.16
Mutilation Anxiety	0.58	0.23
Separation Anxiety	0.46	0.24
Guilt Anxiety	0.91	0.12
Shame Anxiety	0.85	0.29
Diffuse Anxiety	0.85	0.09
Total Anxiety	0.88	0.32
Hostility Outward Overt	0.37	0.62
Hostility Outward Covert	0.27	0.39
Hostility Outward Total	0.27	0.78

Table 2. (Continued)

Scale/Subscale	Multiplier (slope)	Offset (y-intercept)
Hostility Inward	0.54	0.49
Ambivalent Hostility	0.20	0.58
Social Alienation/Personal Disorganization	0.86	-0.03
Cognitive Impairment	0.75	0.02
Health	0.37	0.20
Hopelessness	0.26	0.23
Guilt Depression	0.91	0.12
Shame Depression	0.85	0.29
Hostility Directed Inward	0.54	0.49
Self-Accusation	0.89	0.41
Psychomotor Retardation	0.15	0.25
Somatic Concerns	0.77	0.33
Death Depression	0.92	0.16
Mutilation Depression	0.58	0.23
Death and Mutilation Depression	0.67	0.34
Separation Depression	0.46	0.24
Hostility Outward Overt	0.37	0.62
Hostility Outward Covert	0.27	0.39
Hostility Outward	0.27	0.78
Total Depression	0.77	1.33

Example Calculation

Given a computer-generated score (C), the human equivalent (E) is calculated by multiplying the computer-generated score by the multiplier for the scale or subscale, then adding the offset for the scale or subscale. For example, a computer-generated total anxiety score of 0.54 would be converted as follows: $E = mC + b$; $E = 0.88C + 0.32$; $E = (0.88 * 0.54) + 0.32$; $E = 0.48 + 0.32$; $E = 0.80$.

So, a computer-generated score of 0.54 for total anxiety has a human equivalent score of 0.80.

The norm for total anxiety is 1.48, with a standard deviation of 0.70. The human-equivalent score (0.80) is within one standard deviation of the mean, and thus would be considered to fall within the normal range.

The summaries also indicate to what extent the verbal sample score deviates from the norms that have been obtained for each scale (in terms of standard deviations). PCAD uses the distance of a sample score from the mean for a scale to generate commentary and candidate diagnoses for consideration.

- A score that lies within one standard deviation of the mean is considered "in the normal range."
- A score that is more than one but less than two standard deviations from the mean is "slightly high."

- Between two and three standard deviations, scores are described as "moderately high," and
- Above three standard deviations are described as "very high."

On most scales, PCAD reports only deviations above the mean. Exceptions are Hope, Human Relations, Achievement Strivings, and Quality of Life. For these scales, deviations below the mean are reported as "slightly/moderately/very low."

Finally, the system proposes possible neuropsychiatric diagnoses that the user might consider in evaluating the patient or subject.

Thus, the software system generates four distinct classes of output: (1) an interlinear listing of each grammatical clause and the scores assigned to it; (2) a scoring summary for each content analysis scale, including a comparison to established norms for each scale; (3) an analysis or interpretation, in textual form, of the scale scores; and (4) possible neuropsychiatric diagnostic classifications taken from the *Diagnostic and Statistical Manual,* Fourth Edition of the American Psychiatric Association, 1994, that a clinician might consider in evaluating the subject or patient.

We have adapted the PCAD software to create an initial implementation of a therapeutic agent, called THERAPIST.

THERAPIST begins by presenting a form that the subject can fill out to provide necessary identifying data. The identifying data collected includes: 1. Name. 2. Occupation. 3. Age. 4.Gender. 5. Marital status. 6. Education. 7. Ethnic background. 8. Religion and degree of religious activity (active/inactive). 9. Height. 10.Weight. 11. Number of daughters. 12. Number of sons. 13. Number of brothers.14. Number of sisters.15. Mother's age (or age at death, if deceased). 16. Father's age (or age at death, if deceased). 17. Description of mother's health. 18. Description of father's health. 19. Description of medical illnesses. 20. Description of accidents or injuries. 21. Description of mental illnesses. 22. Description of other health issues. 23. Description of medications taken (name and amount).

In order to obtain an initial understanding of the participant's complaints and worries, the computer program requests that the participant summarize in 100 words or more these complaints, worries, and symptoms. We plan to incorporate introductory comments such as the following to inform potential participants about the nature and goals of this computerized program for psychodynamic psychotherapy.

"Welcome to this program designed to help you understand yourself better. It is organized to compare and contrast your mental and physical status with other people of your sex and age range—children and adult—who are capable of writing about themselves to a computer program and sharing their feelings and attitudes and life problems with an objective artificial intelligence software program that has been intensively researched, scientifically validated, and widely published over many years (www.gb-software.com). The responses and information supplied by participants are regarded as absolutely private and confidential and are not available to anyone other than the participant identifiable only through a password."

"Initially, so you can be personally identified, please provide some personal information regarding your identity, gender, demographic data, past and present physical and mental status, family history, and so forth. This information is used by the computer program to compare the health status of the participant to other participants who were regarded as physically and mentally healthy on the occasions when they provided spoken or written verbal samples over a five-minute period. Their verbal samples were analyzed grammatically clause by clause for the magnitude of over thirty Content Analysis Scales, which have been validated in many books and peer-reviewed scientific journals (Gottschalk and Gleser, 1969; Gottschalk, Lolas, Viney, 1986;William M. Reynolds, 2001; Gottschalk and Bechtel, 1998-2002)."

The longer and more detailed this initial communication is the more reliable the computer program's understanding of the nature and scope of the problems will be. THERAPIST uses the PCAD capability to analyze the semantic content, that is, the meanings, of the verbal text supplied by the participant and to compare the scores obtained from this initial content analysis with the normal scores typically obtained on the Gottschalk-Gleser content analysis scales.

On the basis of the scores obtained from this initial evaluation, the computer program makes responses appropriate to these scores. For example, if all the content analysis scores are not significantly different from the norms for all of these Content Analysis Scales, THERAPIST tells the participant he/she, on the basis of this initial verbal communication, is normal in every respect. If there turns out to be some deviation from the norms—that is, one, two or three standard deviations from the established norm on any of the content analysis scales, THERAPIST communicates this information to the participant in some polite and objective way and, on some occasions, asks the participant for more information or to elaborate on some relevant theme in his/her initial verbal communication.

The following are a number of examples of content analysis outcomes and the corresponding THERAPIST responses that they trigger.

(1) No standard deviations from all the norms. "You certainly are in a happy frame of mind today. I am wondering what is going on in your life that is making you so comfortable and relaxed?"
(2) One standard deviation above the norm for total anxiety only. "I have the feeling that something is worrying you. Would you care to tell me about it?"
(3) Two standard deviations about the norm for total anxiety only. "I get the impression that something is making you feel moderately anxious. Could you elaborate on what is the matter?"
(4) Three standard deviations above the norm for total anxiety only. "Wow! You're certainly very scared about the matter. Tell me more about it."
(5) One standard deviation above the norm for death anxiety only. "The subject of death is on your mind. Tell me more about why you are thinking about death."
(6) Two and three standard deviations above the norm for death anxiety only. "You are certainly preoccupied at this time about dying and death. Tell me more about what is triggering these thought."
(7) One, two or three standard deviation(s) above the norm for mutilation anxiety only. "You are making me aware that you have been thinking about injury and/or damage. Could you elaborate for me why these thoughts are occurring at this time?"
(8) One, two or three standard deviations above the norm for separation anxiety only. "It seems the idea of separation and/or loss worries you. Share with me more about separation, would you?
(9) One, two or three standard deviations above the norm for guilt anxiety only. "You appear to be bothered by guilt feelings. What more do you want to tell me about your guilt feelings?"

(10) One, two or three standard deviations above the norm for shame anxiety only. "You sound like you are embarrassed or ashamed. I wonder whether you have told me all I should know about that in order for me to help you."

(11) One, two or three standard deviations above the norm for diffuse anxiety only. "I recognize you are scared about something disturbing to you. Tell me more so I can understand your situation."

(12) One, two or three standard deviations above the norm for hostility outward (overt or covert). "You are angry and want to retaliate. Please expand and fill out the details so I can better understand how I might help you."

(13) One, two or three standard deviations above the norm for hostility inward only. "You are quite self-critical. How come?"

(14) One, two or three standard deviations above the norm for ambivalent hostility only. "You are telling me that people or something is against you. Maybe hurting you or destroying you."

(15) One, two or three standard deviations above the norm for total depression only. "You seem depressed. How long has your depressed condition been going on and what seems to have precipitated it?"

"Have you consulted a physician, especially a psychiatrist? I strongly recommend that you do so as soon as possible, preferably immediately."

"If you have had any suicidal or homicidal ideas or impulses, you should consult a psychiatrist as soon as possible. Trying to solve such serious problems by a computer program is not possible."

(16) One, two or three standard deviations above the norm for the hopelessness subscale (I) of the Depression Scale. "It sounds as if you have given up hope, that is, that you are feeling hopeless. Am I correct about that? And if so, tell me more about why you feel hopeless."

"Have you consulted a physician, especially a psychiatrist? I strongly recommend that you do so as soon as possible, preferably immediately."

"If you have had any suicidal or homicidal ideas or impulses, you should consult a psychiatrist as soon as possible. Trying to solve such serious problems by a computer program is not possible."

(17) One, two or three standard deviations above the norm for the Self-accusation subscale (II) of the Depression Scale. "Am I to understand that you feel a lot of guilt and shame and are inclined to accuse and disparage yourself. Do you think you are to blame?"

"Have you consulted a physician, especially a psychiatrist? I strongly recommend that you do so as soon as possible, preferably immediately."

"If you have had any suicidal or homicidal ideas or impulses, you should consult a psychiatrist as soon as possible. Trying to solve such serious problems by a computer program is not possible."

(18) One, two or three standard deviations above the norm for the Psychomotor subscale (III) of the Depression Scale. "Do I understand that you are feeling generally retarded and slowed down in action and thinking?"

"Have you consulted a physician, especially a psychiatrist? I strongly recommend that you do so as soon as possible, preferably immediately."

"If you have had any suicidal or homicidal ideas or impulses, you should consult a psychiatrist as soon as possible. Trying to solve such serious problems by a computer program is not possible."

(19) One, two or three standard deviations above the norm for the Somatic concerns subscale (IV) of the Depression Scale. "You are telling me that you have some bodily malfunctioning, maybe have some problem sleeping and maybe some sexual disturbance? Would you kindly elaborate?"
"Have you consulted a physician, especially a psychiatrist? I strongly recommend that you do so as soon as possible, preferably immediately."
"If you have had any suicidal or homicidal ideas or impulses, you should consult a psychiatrist as soon as possible. Trying to solve such serious problems by a computer program is not possible."

(20) One, two or three standard deviations above the norm for the Death and Mutilation depression subscale (V) of the Depression Scale. "Do you mean to tell me that you are worried about being injured or dying? I wonder why fear is consuming you? What has happened that causes you to have such preoccupations?"
"Have you consulted a physician, especially a psychiatrist? I strongly recommend that you do so as soon as possible, preferably immediately."
"If you have had any suicidal or homicidal ideas or impulses, you should consult a psychiatrist as soon as possible. Trying to solve such serious problems by a computer program is not possible."

(21) One, two or three standard deviations above the norm for the Separation depression subscale (VI) of the Depression Scale. "Do you feel that you have you been deserted, abandoned or ostracized? Did something happen in your life in which you feel you have lost support? Or are those events just a threat or a bad memory?"
"Have you consulted a physician, especially a psychiatrist? I strongly recommend that you do so as soon as possible, preferably immediately."
"If you have had any suicidal or homicidal ideas or impulses, you should consult a psychiatrist as soon as possible. Trying to solve such serious problems by a computer program is not possible."

(22) One, two or three standard deviations above the norm for the Hostility Outward depression subscale (VII) of the Depression Scale. "So you are mad at others and you notice others tend to hurt others? Tell me more about your self in these regards.
"Have you consulted a physician, especially a psychiatrist? I strongly recommend that you do so as soon as possible, preferably immediately."
"If you have had any suicidal or homicidal ideas or impulses, you should consult a psychiatrist as soon as possible. Trying to solve such serious problems by a computer program is not possible."

(23) One, two or three standard deviations above the norm for the Social Alienation-Personal Disorganization Scale. "I wonder whether you ever hear voices or see things that other people do not. Or whether you feel people are talking or thinking bad things about you. Or whether you actually feel a bit disorganized. In any event tell me more about these matters.
"Have you consulted a physician, especially a psychiatrist? I strongly recommend that you do so as soon as possible, preferably immediately."

"If you have had any suicidal or homicidal ideas or impulses, you should consult a psychiatrist as soon as possible. Trying to solve such serious problems by a computer program is not possible."

(24) One, two or three standard deviations above the norm for the Cognitive and Intellectual Impairment Scale only. "Do you have some trouble with your recent memories, for example, where you put some things or where you are or the names of family members or friends? Or do you feel you are just as sharp intellectually as you ever have been?"

(25) One, two or three standard deviations below the norm for the Hope Scale only. "Do you feel as positive and optimistic as ever? Are people giving you the help or support to which you are accustomed? Or you feel downright hopeless? Please tell me more about your level of hopefulness."

(26) One, two or three standard deviations below the norm for the Human Relations Scale only. "From what you have communicated to me, I have the impression that the quality of your relationships with others is not going so well. Could you give me more details so that I could understand the bases for the difficulties you are having? I am hoping I can help you."

(27) One, two or three standard deviations below the norm on the Achievement Strivings Scale. "I believe you are telling me that you are having some problems in achieving some of your aims and goals. Would you tell me more about these problems so that I understand them better and so I can be of possible usefulness in helping you satisfy some of your achievement strivings."

(28) One, two or three standard deviations above the norms on the Health and Health/Sickness Scale. "I gather from your messages to me that you are troubled by some kind of illness which interferes with your health and well-being. Can you tell me more about the trouble you are having?"

"Do you have a family practitioner, internist, or medical specialist? If not, I recommend that you obtain such a physician right away."

(29) One, two or three standard deviations above the norms for Dependency and Dependency Frustration Scales. "I think you have communicated to me that there are some shortcomings in the satisfaction of your dependency needs. Could you tell me more about your normal dependency and the frustrations you are having of your dependent needs."

(30) One, two or three standard deviations below the norms on the Quality of Life Scale. "I get the impression from your messages to me that the quality of your life is not very good. So that I can understand your life situation better, would you tell me more about what is going on in your life in this respect."

(31) One, two or three standard deviations above the norms for the Total Anxiety Scale and the Depression Scale or some abnormal score in other Content Scale, such as the Quality of Life Scale or the Human Relations Scale or one of the Hostility Scales. "It sounds to me that you may have a depression with some anxiety or maybe occasional panic states. Have you been getting some professional help for this disorder or have you been suffering in silence? Tell me more about your self."

(32) One, two or three standard deviations above the norms on the Social Alienation-Personal Disorganization and other relevant Content Analysis Scales, such as, the Hostility Scales, the Anxiety Scales, the Human Relations Scale, the Achievement

Strivings Scale, the Health/Sickness Scales. "I gather from what you tell me that you have been experiencing some very uncomfortable mental symptoms. Can you tell me more about your self? And have you been getting some professional help for your condition?"

(33) One, two or three standard deviations above the norms for the Cognitive and Intellectual Impairment Scale as well as any other Content Analysis Scale or Scales. "I wonder whether you are having any problems focusing your attention or experiencing some troubles with your memory. If so, how long have you had these symptoms? And are you getting any professional help for these difficulties? Tell me more about your self."

(34) One, two or three standard deviations above the norms for two or more Content Analysis Scales. "These are matters we need to talk about more. There must have been a number of stressors in your life that bring on such mental strain. I believe we should consider communicating regularly--maybe daily or weekly--to help me understand the tough times you have gone through. I believe that communicating with someone else about these events will help relieve the inner pressures you are experiencing. Also, I wonder whether your family doctor is prescribing some medications for you that might relieve some of your symptoms. And if so, what are they? Can you give me the names of the drugs, how often you take them and what the doses are?"

(35) One, two or three standard deviations above the norms for any Content Analysis Scales. "Thanks for confiding in me. You can contact me whenever you want to do so. As you know, to contact me you have to first submit your password so that our communications are confidential and attributed only to you and me."

At this point, we have the beginning of a fruitful conversation between THERAPIST and the participant who, at will, can share more information with THERAPIST, which THERAPIST is likely to respond to in a supportive and sometimes inquiring manner.

The computer program has an excellent memory, and it will keep track of the participant's identification, present and past history, family history, mental and physical status, and it will keep a good and reliable record of all the preceding communications between the participant and itself. On some occasions where appropriate, THERAPIST may well refer to some of the information retained in its memory and remind the participant about these past intercommunications.

THERAPIST will always be interested in responding to verbal communications from the participant on a regular basis. Like any psychodynamic psychotherapist, THERAPIST is ready to work with the participant on any ramifications of the initial problems that were shared or new ones.

THERAPIST has the ability to help understand and analyze dreams if the participant recalls them and can free-associate about details in the dreams.

We have faced several interesting challenges in adapting the PCAD software to the interactivity required by THERAPIST. While PCAD is useful in a psychiatry or psychology research setting, for example in exploring the writings of the Unabomber for evidence of psychopathology (Gottschalk and Gottschalk, 1999), or in predicting the outcome of psychiatric commitment hearings (Lavid et al, 2002), it is strongly oriented to the analysis of samples that are larger than many conversational utterances. For reliable results, the recommended minimum input sample length is 80 words. The focus is usually on overall scale scores, aggregated over all the clauses in a sample, because at that level the established norms can be used for comparison purposes.

At least two earlier efforts have been made to apply the PCAD scoring software in interaction settings. In the first (Gottschalk et al, 2003), the software was used to analyze utterances in dialogues among medical personnel and families of patients in a surgical intensive care unit. The problem of short utterances was addressed by aggregating utterances by speaker, enabling calculation of both a per-utterance and cumulative sample score for each speaker. The second interaction application was in a commercial web-based system that generates responses to subject entries, similar in spirit to the original Eliza (Weizenbaum, 1966), but with the (pre-written) response determined by the content analysis scores on the various scales (Journal Genie, 2004).

We are aware that having to type into a computer, at this point in the English language and with fairly good spelling, presents some constraints to our goals. The goals of THERAPIST are to read what the patient writes, decide whether what the patient says has any adverse neuropsychiatric characteristics, has any normal neuropsychiatric dimensions, has any positive and healthy features, decides what the various combinations of these dimensions are with respect to one individual, aims to alleviate the discomfort and disabilities currently involving this individual to any extent possible, and invite the individual to share his mental and emotional experiences through the medium of verbal behavior.

The detection and measurement capability of our existing verbal sample scoring software supplies a useful starting point for our goal of therapeutic support, but it is only a small fraction of what would be needed to attempt psychotherapy. We are in the process of adding entity recognition and tracking to the core content analysis results to better establish the context in which emotions and mental processes of interest appear. For example, if hostility outward is consistently detected with respect to a particular individual, interaction may be guided to examine that relationship in greater depth.

Before a dialogue system such as THERAPIST can respond to mental processes and emotions, it must detect them. Psychiatry and psychology have long experience in the definition, detection, and measurement of these phenomena, both in characterizing the people in whom they occur, their associated behaviors, their diagnostic classification, and in selecting and measuring the efficacy of therapeutic interventions. Our use of the Gottschalk-Gleser content analysis scales provides a means of detecting meaningful psychobiological content in linguistic behaviors, and such information provides cues and guidelines for psychotherapeutic interaction.

Additional work will be needed in a variety of areas before we can offer readily and easily usable computerized software that can provide diagnostic medical and neuropsychiatric information that can serve as a basis for psychotherapeutic involvement. Systematic responses by THERAPIST will need greater flexibility than has been available in our current text template approach. On the dialogue level, we need to incorporate the medical and neuropsychiatric assessment within a user model, and create a model of the psychotherapy process that can be used to drive a dialogue move engine, such as, TrindiKit (Larsson and Traum, 2000). The need for interacting functionality at so many levels suggests that psychotherapy offers a fertile ground for further work in dialogue research.

To enhance the relationship between the subject (computer software user) and the computer software program (derived in part from PCAD—psychiatric content analysis and diagnosis), we are changing the name THERAPIST to the name FRIEND, which we hope to some extent will be valid.

The question is certainly fair to ask how effective computerized psychotherapy can be. There is considerable published research on the efficacy of psychotherapy. Rosenzweig (1936) was a pioneer in pointing out that there were implicit common factors in diverse methods of psychotherapy. Luborsky (1995), in a creative and clever paper, observed more precisely that there were common factors across different psychotherapies—such as, the attention of a therapist who has a convincing allegiance to the beneficial values of the therapy being provided, the scheduled opportunity to articulate and verbalize one's personal life history and experiences, and the recurring occasions to share private mental conflicts and symptoms. Luborsky, with regards to the issue of the relative outcomes of psychotherapies, repeated Rosenzweig's quote from Alice in Wonderland: "everybody has won, so all shall have prizes" which was the "Dodo bird's verdict" after judging the race. The "Dodo bird verdict" has become commonly used in clinical research examining the differential effects of various psychotherapies and/or belief systems. No one has systematically tested the efficacy of computerized psychotherapy, but that activity should be soon forthcoming. A more recent publication by Luborsky and his collaborators (Luborsky et al., 2002), examines17 meta-analyses of comparisons of active treatments with each other, in contrast to the more usual comparisons of active treatment with controls, a paper which addresses relevant questions possibly raised by any readers of this article.

Conclusions

A computerized neuropsychiatric diagnostic and psychodynamic psychotherapeutic procedure is described. The scientific foundations and published pertinent research on which this methodology is based are cited and reviewed, including some previous clinical trials.

The potential diagnostic and therapeutic usefulness of this unique computerized technological achievement are suggested as a therapeutic adjuvant or instrument. Its limitations are noted, especially with respect to use with persons who have disabling medical disorders and who are experiencing suicidal and/or homicidal ideation.

Further development and testing of this computer software are in progress.

References

American Psychiatric Association. *Diagnostic and Statistical Manual.* Fourth Edition. American Psychiatric Press. 1994.

Bechtel R. Developments in computer science with applications in text analysis. In Carl W. Roberts (Ed.) *Text Analysis for the Social Sciences. Methods for Drawing Statistical Inferences from Texts and Transcripts.* Mahway, New Jersey: Lawrence Erlbaum Associates, 239-250, 1997.

Bechtel RJ and Gottschalk LA. Detection of neuropsychiatric states of interest in text. AAAI Fall Symposium on Dialogue Systems for Health Communication. *American Association for Artificial Intelligence,* October 2004.

Gleser GC, Winget C, Seligman, Rauh JL. Evaluation of psychotherapy in with adolescents using content analysis of verbal samples. In: LA Gottschalk (Ed.) *The Content Analysis of Verbal Samples: Further Studies. (pp.* 213-233) New York: Spectrum, 1979.

Gottschalk LA. Depressions—psychodynamic considerations. In: JE Cole and JR Wittenborn (Eds.) *Pharmacotherapy of Depressions* (pp. 30-46). Springfield, Ill. Charles C Thomas, 1966.

Gottschalk LA. A hope scale applicable to verbal samples. *Archives of General Psychiatry.* 30:779-785, 1974.

Gottschalk LA. (Ed.) *The Content Analysis of Verbal Behavior. Further Studies.* New York: Spectrum Publications. 1979.

Gottschalk LA. Content Analysis of Verbal Behavior. *New Findings and Clinical Applications.* Hillsdale, New Jersey: Lawrence Erlbaum Publisher. 1995.

Gottschalk LA, The unobstrusive measurement of psychological states and traits. In: Carl W. Roberts (Ed.). *Text Analysis for the Social Sciences. Methods for Drawing Statistical Inferences from Texts and Transcripts.* Mahway, New Jersey: Lawrence Erlbaum Associates, pp. 117-130, 1997.

Gottschalk LA, The application of a computerized measurement of the content analysis of natural language to the assessment of the effects of psychoactive.drugs. *Methods and Findings in Experimental and Clinical Pharmacology.* 21: 133-138, 1999.

Gottschalk LA, The application of computerized content analysis of natural language in psychotherapy research now and in the future. *American Journal of Psychotherapy.* 54:305-311, 2000.

Gottschalk LA and Bechtel RJ. The measurement of anxiety through the computer analysis of verbal samples. *Comprehensive Psychiatry:* 23:4 (July/August). 1982.

Gottschalk LA and Bechtel RJ, Artificial intelligence and the computerization of the content analysis of natural language. *Artificial Intelligence in Medicine.* 1:131-111, 1989.

Gottschalk LA and Bechtel RJ, *Psychologic and Neuropsychiatric Assessment Survey: Computerized Content Analysis of Natural Language or Verbal Texts.* Palo Alto: California: Mind Garden (3803 East Bayshore Road, Palo Alto, CA, 943031), 1993.

Gottschalk LA and Bechtel R. Computerized measurement of the content analysis of natural language for use in biomedical and neuropsychiatric research, *Computer Methods and Programs in Biomedicine:* 47:123-130. 1995.

Gottschalk LA and Bechtel RJ, PCAD 2000—*Psychiatric Content Analysis and Diagnosis.* Corona del Mar, CA: GB Software (4607 Perham Road; Corona del Mar, CA 92625), 1998-2003.

Gottschalk LA, Bechtel RJ, Buchman TA, Ray SE. Computerized content analysis of conversational interactions. *CIN: Computers, Informatics, Nursing.* 21:249-258. 2003.

Gottschalk LA, Bechtel RJ, Buchman TA, Ray SE. A computerized measure of quality of life derived from the content analysis of natural language. *Research Communications in Biological Psychology and Psychiatry.* 27:3-14, 2003(b).

Gottschalk LA, Bechtel RJ, Buchman TA, Ray SE. Measurement of hope and associated neuropsychiatric dimensions by the computerized content analysis of speech and verbal texts. In: Jacklin Elliott (Ed.) *Interdisciplinary Perspectives on Hope.* Nova Science Publishers. (pp.205-220), 2004.

Gottschalk LA, Bechtel RJ, Maguire GA, Harrington DE, Levinson D, Franklin DL, Caracamo D. Computerized measurement of cognitive impairment and associated neuropsychiatric dimensions. *Comprehensive Psychiatry*. 41:326-333, 2000.

Gottschalk LA, Bechtel RJ, Maguire GA, Katz M, Levinson DM, Harrington DE, Nakamura K, Franklin DL. Computerized detection of cognitive impairment and associated neuropsychiatric dimensions from the content analysis of verbal samples. *American Journal of Drug and Alcohol Abuse*. 28:653-668, 2002.

Gottschalk LA, DeFrancisco D, Bechtel RJ. Computerized content analysis of some adolescent writings of Napoleon Bonaparte. A test of the validity of the method. *Journal of Nervous and Mental Disease*. 190:542-548, 2002.

Gottschalk LA, Fronczek J, Abel L, Buchsbaum MS, Fallon JH. The neurobiology of anxiety, anxiety-displacement, and anxiety denial. *Psychotherapy and Psychosomatics*. 70:17-24, 2001.

Gottschalk LA and Gleser GC. *The Measurement of Psychological States Through the Content Analysis of Verbal Behavior*. Berkeley, Los Angeles: California: The University of California Press. 1969.

Gottschalk LA and Gottschalk LH. Computerized content analysis of the Unabomber's writings. *American Journal of Forensic Psychiatry*. 20:5-31. 1999.

Gottschalk, LA, Hausmann, C, Brown, JS. A computerized scoring system for use with content analysis scales. *Comprehensive Psychiatry*. 16:77-90, 1975.

Gottschalk LA, Holcombe R, Jackson D, Bechtel RJ. The effects of anticancer chemotherapeutic drugs upon cognitive function and other neuropsychiatric dimensions in breast cancer patients. *Methods and Findings in Experimental and Clinical Pharmacology*. 25:117-122, 2003.

Gottschalk LA, Lolas F, Viney LL. (Eds.). *Content Analysis of Verbal Behavior. Significance in Clinical Medicine and Psychiatry*. Berlin, Heidelberg, New York, Tokyo: Springer-Verlag, 1986.

Gottschalk LA, Winget CN, *Gleser GC. Manual of Instructions for Using the Gottschalk-Gleser Content Analysis Scales: Anxiety, Hostility, Social Alienation-Personal Disorganization.* Los Angeles, Berkeley, University of California Press. 1969.

Guinn C and Hubal R. Extracting emotional information from the text of spoken dialog. *Proceedings of the International Conference on User Modeling Workshop, Assessing and Adapting to User Attitudes and Affect: Why, When and How?,* June 22, 2003, Pittsburgh, PA. 2003.

Journal Genie website. http://www.journalgenie.com/ 2004.

Koch U and Schofer G (Hrsg.). Sprachinhaltsanalyse in der psychosomatiscshen und psychiatrischen Forschung. *Grundlagen und Anwendungsstudien mit den Affektskalen von Gottschalk und Gleser.* Weinheim und Munchen: Psychologie Verlags Union, 1986.

Larsson S and Traum D. Information state and dialogue management in the TRINDI dialogue move engine toolkit. In *Natural Language Engineering Special Issue on Best Practice in Spoken Language Dialogue Systems Engineering,* pp. 323-340. Cambridge University Press, U.K. 2000.

Lavid NR, Grayden TJ, Gottschalk LA, Bechtel RJ. Computerized assessment of the enforced hospitalization and medication from notes of hospitalized psychiatric inpatients. *American Journal of Forensic Psychiatry*. 23:55-69, 2002.

Liu H, Lieberman H, and Selker T. A model of textual affect sensing using real-world knowledge. *Proceedings of the 2003 International Conference on Intelligent User Interfaces,* IUI 2003, pp.125-132. January 12-15, 2003, Miami, FL. 2003.

Luborsky L. Are common factors across different psychotherapies the main explanation for the Dodo bird verdict that "Everyone has won so all shall have prizes"? *Clinical Psychology: Science and Practice,* 2:106-109, 1995.

Luborsky L, Rosenthal R, Diguer L, Andrusyna TP, Berman JS, Levitt JT, Seligman DA, Krause ED. The Dodo bird verdict is alive and well—mostly. *Clinical Psychology: Science and Practice.* 9:2-12, 2002.

Madden S. WebEvaluator: deducing emotion and personality from web pages. http://www.cs.berkeley.edu/~madden/WebEvaluator/WebEvaluator.htm. 1999.

Maguire GA, Gottschalk LA, Riley GD, Franklin DL, Bechtel RJ, Ashurst J. Stuttering: Neuropsychiatric features measured by the content analysis of speech and the effect of risperidone on stuttering severity. *Comprehensive Psychiatry.* 40:308-314, 1999.

Reynolds WM. Psychiatric Content Analysis and Diagnosis (PCAD 2000). Barbara S. Plake, James C. Impara, Linda L. Murphy (Eds.) *The Fourteenth Mental Measurements Yearbook.* The University of Nebraska Press, 2001.

Rosenzweig S. Some implicit common factors in diverse methods of psychotherapy. *American Journal of Orthopsychiatry.* 6:412-415, 1936.

Subasic P. Affect analysis of text using fuzzy semantic typing. *The Sixth ACM SIGKDD International Conference on Knowledge Discovery and Data Mining.* Boston, August 20-23, 2000.

Weizenbaum J. ELIZA - A computer program for the study of natural language communication between man and machine. *Communications of the ACM,* 9:36-45. 1966.

Winget C, Seligman R, Rauh RL, Gleser GC. Social alienation-personal disorganization assessment in disturbed and normal adolescents. *Journal of Nervous and Mental Disease.* 167:282-287, 1979.

Zhe Z and Boucouvalas AC. Text-to-emotion engine for real time Internet communication." *International Symposium on Communication Systems, Networks and DSPs*, pp. 164-168. 15-17 July 2002, Staffordshire University, UK. 2002.

OTHER NEUROPSYCHIATRIC RESEARCH OF INTEREST

To illustrate some of the other kinds of content analysis research in which I have been involved, I have selected several representative examples. In 1974 I published a paper entitled "A hope scale applicable to verbal samples" (Gottschalk, LA. 1974) which had two main purposes: 1. to carry out a preliminary set of construct validation studies using the Hope Scale; 2. and to obtain norms for Hope scale scores and intecorrelations with scores for other psychological states. Construct validation studies indicated significant negative correlations between Hope scale scores and psychiatric ratings on the Brief Psychiatric Rating Scale for Depression and the Anergic factor scores, on the Hamilton Depression Rating scale factors of Anxiety-Depression and Sleep Disturbance, and also with scores from the Jacobs Ego Weakness scale. Significant positive results occurred with scores from the Anant Belongingness scale. Hope scores were found capable of predicting favorable outcome among patients going to a Mental Health Crisis Clinic, patients likely to follow neuropsychiatric treatment recommendations, the survival time for patients with terminal cancer, and the degree of improvement in the Depression factor of the Brief Psychiatric Rating scale in acute schizophrenic patients after a single dose of a tranquilizer (thioridazine). Percentile Hope scores were obtained from a normatrive sample of children (N=109), adults (N=91), and a group of psychiatric outpatients (N=68).

In 1977 with colleagues (Gottschalk, Aronow, Prakash, 1977)? studied the effects of marijuana and placebo-marijuana smoking on the psychological states and psychophysiological cardiovascular functioning in anginal patients. Specifically, male anginal patients with angiographically documented coronary artery disease, in a randomized double-blind cross overstudy, smoked one marijuana cigarette (containing 18 mg. tetrahydrocannabinol [THC]) on one morning and one placebo marijuana cigarette (containing 0.05 mg THC) on a successive morning. Significant increases occurred in average cognitive and intellectual impairment scores, derived from the objective content analysis of five minutes of speech obtained from these patients, 30 minutes after smoking the marijuana cigarette as compared to smoking the placebo marijuana. The cognitive impairment scores decreased to near pre-smoking levels 60 minutes after smoking. No significant average changes occurred in anxiety or three hostility scales (hostility outward, hostility inward, ambivalent hostility) following smoking marijuana. Sizeable individual differences were noted in the psychological responses to marijuana smoking, due presumably to personality differences and/or differences in THC pharmacokinetics. Significant psychocardiovascular hemodynamic correlations, as measured by echocardiography, were observed during placebo-marijuana smoking between hostility inward scores and systolic blood pressure and ejection fraction, between overt hostility outward scores and diastolic blood pressure, and between anxiety scores and stroke volume and left ventricular end-diastolic dimension and left ventricular diastolic volume. *These significant psychophysiological correlations were all eliminated during marijuana smoking.* In view of associated findings that marijuana smoking decreases myocardial oxygen delivery, decreased exercise time until the onset of anginal pain, and increased myocardial demand in anginal patients, *the use of marijuana by anginal patients is clearly inadvisable.*

In 1981 I was invited to contribute a paper at a Symposium, held at the Casa de Maria, on Creativity sponsored jointly by the Institute of Religious Studies and the Department of German and Slavic Languages and Literature, University of California at Santa Barbara. I described, at that time, what I thought were the major characteristics of creativity: (1) originality and uniqueness; (2) comprehensibility to others; (3) utility; (4) generalizability to allied and other fields; (5) a capacity for continued and repeated creative outputs in similar and/or different fields; and (6) a capacity to stimulate others to artistic, literary, or scientific originality. Whereas, there is limited current knowledge of hereditary factors contributing to creativity—intelligence certainly plays a role, there are familial and environmental factors that are definitely influential. With regards to the development of creative prowess in children, it is helpful temporarily to preserve and encourage the use of primary-process thinking (that is, obscuring the differences in time, place, and person) so that this mental activity (primary process) can be called upon and reflected about at will. The demonstration of creative ability in parental, kinship, and social networks needs to be exposed to young people. That is, the effects of kinship creativity catalyzing creative motivations in family members and exposure to other creative people are key factors. The encouragement of analogical thinking and imagination in children and the capacity to turn on and off such mental activity by secondary-process (differentiating) thinking is useful. Artistic and scientific creativity have features in common and situational or everyday creativity, though short-term, can be reflected in more long-term behavior.

In 1980 a study was made of the relationship of aging and its assessment with the Cognitive Impairment scale (Gottschalk, Cohn, Terman, Wolf, 1980) . Based on the frequency of use of selected verbal content categories—in a clinical trial involving patients with senile dementia—a group of elderly individuals (N= 38) was investigated. They ranged in age from 60 to 80 years of age and showed evidence of moderate impairment of cognitive function on a clinical assessment measure (the Sandoz Clinical Assessment-Geriatrics [SCAG] Shader et al., 1974) . A five-minute speech sample was obtained from each member of the group by purposely ambiguous instructions to talk about any interesting or dramatic life experiences. These patients showed significantly higher scores ($t=3.48$; $p<.001$) on the Gottschalk Cognitive Impairment scale applied to their speech samples (mean=1.6; SD=1.8) than a younger (mean age 30.6 years) group (N=58) of adults (mean=0.43; SD=1.25).

In 1983, Gottschalk, Eckardt, Pautler, and Wolf published a paper summarizing the correlations between scores obtained from 18 commonly used neuropsychological tests and 13 weighted verbal categories from the Gottschalk Cognitive Impairment scale. This study has contributed to the validation of this Cognitive Impairment scale.

At the request of Gannett publications in Washington, D.C., the Cognitive Impairment scale was applied to the transcripts of the extemporaneous speeches given by the two presidential candidates during their 1980 (Reagan and Carter) and 1984 (Reagan and Mondale) televised debates (Gottschalk, Uliana, Gilbert, 1988). One presidential candidate (Ronald Reagan) was found to have significantly higher cognitive impairment scores during these debates than the other presidential candidate, and the cognitive impairment scores derived from Ronald Reagan's verbal behavior became progressively more elevated over the period from his debates with Carter (1980) to those with Mondale (1984). The authors commented that "in addition to the general medical examination, which top political officials undergo as an informal condition for public office, periodic neuropsychiatric examinations are technically feasible, whether or not requiring these is politically possible"(p.613).

In a series of studies (Gottschalk, Fronczek, Abel, Buchsbaum, Fallon, 2001), my colleagues and I examined the relationship of the verbal expression of anxiety, anxiety-displacement, and anxiety-denial to the concomitant cerebral neurobiology of localized cerebral glucose metabolic rates as measured by PET (positron emission tomography) scanning. We had previously demonstrated from the anxiety scores, derived from the content analysis of speech of normal individuals, that these anxiety scores occurring in the dreams identified by the subject's rapid eye movement (REM) sleep were significantly intercorrelated with glucose metabolic rate in different brain areas in comparison to when the anxiety scores were obtained from mental experiences reported (after awakening) during non-REM sleep or during wakeful mentation.

The purpose of these studies was to examine the intercorrelations found between anxiety attributed to the self, anxiety-displacement, and anxiety-denial measured from computerized content analysis of five-minute verbal reports of subjective thoughts and feelings obtained from wakeful subjects and localized cerebral glucose metabolic rates during PET scanning. The subjects were 10 wakeful young healthy males. Their anxiety scores were derived from computerized content analysis of five minute reports they gave during a 30 minute period following an intravenous injection of F D-deoxyglucose (FDG). The subjects were moved 32-45 minutes after this injection to obtain a PET scan which records all of the localized cerebral glucose metabolic rates during the 30 minutes following the FDG injection.

Significant intercorrelations of localized cerebral glucose metabolic rates with scores of self-anxiety, anxiety-displacement, and anxiety-denial were found in dissimilar brain locations depending on the type of anxiety involved. The significant correlations occurred in brain regions known to be involved with the functions of emotions, cognition, and vision. Clearly, specific combinations of cerebral areas, based on glucose metabolic rates, are associated with different verbal expressions of anxiety.

The current use of Adderall (a combination of amphetamine salts) in the treatment of Attention Deficit Disorder (ADD) was forshadowed by research of Gottschalk and associates (Gottschalk, Bates, Waskow, Katz, Olson, 1971) who found that amphetamine significantly increased scores derived from the content analysis of five-minute speech samples on an Achievement Strivings scale; whereas chlorpromazine had no such effect.

BIBLIOGRAPHY

Louis A. Gottschalk. Psychoanalytic contributions to the generation of creativity in children. *Psychiatry.* 44:210-229, 1981.

Louis A. Gottschalk. The application of a computerized measurement of the content analysis of natural language to the assessment of psychoactive drugs. *Methods and Findings in Experimental and Clinical Pharmacology.* 21:133-138, 1999.

Louis A. Gottschalk, Wilbert S. Aronow, Ravi Prakash. Effect of marihuana and placebo-marihuana smoking on psychological state and on psychophysiological cardiovascular function in anginal patients. *Biological Psychiatry.* 12:255-266, 1977.

Louis A. Gottschalk, DE Bates, IE Waskow, MM Katz, and J Olson. Effect of amphetamine or chlorpromazine on achievement strivinbgs derived from the content analysis of speech, *Comprehensive Psychiatry.* 12;430-435, 1971.

Louis A. Gottschalk, Michael J. Eckardt, Jay Cohn, Stanley J. Terman, Robert J. Wolf. A cognitive impairment scale applicable to verbal samples and its possible use in clinical trials in patients with dementia. *Psychopharmacology Bulletin.* 16: 25-27, 1980.

Louis A. Gottschalk, Michael J. Eckardt, C.P. Pautler, Robert J. Wolf, Stanley J. Terman. Cognitive impairment derived from verbal samples. *Comprehensive Psychiatry.* 24:6-19, 1983.

Louis A. Gottschalk, Janny Fronczek, Lennart Abel, Monte S. Buchsman, James H. Fallon. The neurobiology of anxiety, anxiety-displacement, and anxiety-denial. *Psychotherapy and Psychosomatics.* 70:17-24, 2001.

Louis A. Gottschalk and Leah H. Gottschalk. Computerized content analysis of the Unabomber's writings. *American Journal of Forensic Psychiatry.* 20:5-31, 1999.

Louis A. Gottschalk, Regina Uliana, Rhonda Gilbert. Presidential candidates and cognitive impairment measured from behavior in campaign debates. *Public Administration Review.* 48:613-619, 1988.

MEMOIRS OF MY MOTHER

My mother was very unusual. She obviously loved boys. She had four sons and no daughters. We were about three years apart in birth. I was the third son. My oldest brother was Max Jules. His nickname was "Buzzie". My next brother was Edmond. He had a number of nicknames, and I will mention some of them. One of them was "Blackadoiey;" he had black hair, and the rest of us had lighter hair. I suppose he got the name from my parents because he looked like a little blackberry when he was an infant. And another nickname was "Desperado." I was told by my mother that he was given the latter name because he resembled a comic strip character named "Desperate Ambrose." Edmond occasionally had temper tantrums, which must have gotten him this name. And he often talked in his sleep; I know because I slept with him for many years when I was a boy. I was named Louis, and sometimes my father called me "Ludie." My youngest brother was Charles. His only nickname was "Charlie." My parents forgot to give him a middle name, and he wanted one like the rest of us. So he gave himself the middle name of Robert.

My earliest memory of my mother (See beginning section, p. 1-EARLY MEMORIES) was revealed to me in a dream that I had while training to be a psychoanalyst at the Institute for Psychoanalysis in Chicago, where I was also in a residency in Child Psychiatry at Michael Reese Hospital. My training analyst was a famous pediatrician and a psychoanalyst by the name of George Mohr. While in psychoanalysis with him, I had a dream in which a little baby was climbing some huge stairs. These stairs had a carpet on them, and there was some kind of pattern in the carpet that the baby could see. On the first landing of these stairs there was a stained-glass window. As he went further up the stairs, there was-of all things-on the second floor, a kitchen. This baby was barely managing being able to get up these huge stairs. And they were huge' The baby was trying to restrain a cry. When he finally got into the kitchen, he vaguely saw in the background his mother, and he started to cry out for her. He had a brief glimpse of his father standing near his mother.

It was clear that I was the baby in this dream and that the baby's perception of the carpeted stairs, the stained-glass window on the first landing of the staircase, the kitchen on the second floor, and other dream details were forgotten childhood perceptions that were recalled and flashed back into the dream scene The emotions the baby was experiencing were emotions that at one time during my infancy I had experienced. Just recalling this dream, while in my analysis, I would get a strong feeling of anxiety. I would also get some transient hives, also known medically as urticaria. Also, recalling this dream picture, many years after having the dream, could make my heart rate accelerate to over 115-120 beats per minute.

The dream was triggered by the phase of the analysis in which I was, but also by a dream stimulus of unjustifiable adverse criticism by a psychoanalytic supervisor of my psychoanalytic treatment of a patient with ulcerative colitis. Apparently this dream stimuli elicited an old real memory of my looking for my mother. My mother was still alive at the time that I was having my personal psychoanalysis, and I asked her about some of the details that occurred in the dream. She informed me that there was such a house in which we lived. It was in st. Louis, Missouri, on Lucas Avenue. Apparently, several families were living in this house, my maternal grandparents, I gather, my own parents and their children, and my uncle Louis and aunt Annie Mutrux, with their budding family. Apparently, there was a kitchen on the second floor in the portion of the house where my own parents lived. (My brother Charlie was born later when we lived at 7416 Washington in St.Louis, Missouri). In any event , talking about this dream with my mother, she informed me that when I was a baby, her father, Jules Mutrux, had just passed away. I must have been, at that time, about six months of age, for I learned recently that he died on January 10, 1917, and I was born on August 26, 1916.

I suppose that she was grief-stricken and temporarily, perhaps, not entirely accessible to me to the degree I desired.

The next memories of my mother, memories that are much easier to retrieve, are memories that date from our living at 7416 Washington in University City, Missouri, a suburb of St. Louis. This was a beautiful house, and I have visited there several times since moving way from St. Louis in 1946 to serve in the United States Public Health Service during World War II, for it is still standing. I can remember sleeping in a large bedroom on the second floor. I think my father had a room on the second floor, too. Mother , I believe, sometimes slept with us or with me, and sometimes I think we had separate beds in the front of the house in a large bedroom.

I remember that we had a forest behind us, which was full of large trees and bushes and little wild animals. We also had a chicken house and some chickens. And I remember, as a little boy, probably four or five years of age, going into that chicken house and looking, with considerable curiosity at those chickens. Once I got too close to a chicken and the rooster of the hen house flew up at me and pecked me on the face, on my left cheek. I had a scar for many years after that.

Across the street from our house there lived a family with a girl by the name of Cynthia. Although it must have been very young for me, I remember being fascinated with Cynthia and having a feeling of great attraction to her. I can rather remember her face and her appearance and her wearing a light lavender dress. I think I was invited to a birthday party for her, and that was a big occasion.

My brothers and I had a lot of fun. I remember that we played together, and we got along well. I had this older brother, Edmond. And then this younger brother, Charlie, came along. We were very good friends. I remember a Christmas and my oldest brother, Max Jules, saying "Do you hear that noise on the roofl? That's Santa Claus getting ready to come down the chimney." I couldn't imagine a red-dressed Santa Claus with a big white beard coming down the chimney and not getting burned and not getting his hair and white beard very sooty. My other brother, Jules, seemed very serious about this. So I rather assumed that his story about Santa coming down the chimney was true.

I remember that my father was often playing the violin or the piano and that he had many musician and artist friends around the house. I remember sitting in the kitchen one day and my father was talking to a group of his friends about how capable his children were. At that age, I had not learned how to write my name (or write anything for that matter). But when my father or one of the other men, who was talking about some great authors, had asked could I write, I said "Sure". So I scribbled several pages of script on a piece of paper. And then they asked me to read what I had written. I must have been about four or five years of age. So I looked at this writing and was momentarily embarrassed. But I noted that my mother, especially, and other elders had also read script that looked unintelligible to me. So I just made up a story, reading my scribbles and telling some kind of yarn. The grown-ups said it was very good! I wish, now, I could remember what that story was that I read. This must have been one of the earliest projective tests that has ever occurred. My father and those other gentlemen were so considerate and kind not to laugh at my creative efforts. This episode happened about 86 years ago. I wonder whether that little experience contributed to my love of writing.

My mother always seemed available to us and very patient with us boys. Before I go into detail to share some of these experiences with you, let me digress a moment to tell you first about my maternal grandmother.

I can remember my maternal grandmother, for though she did not live with us, she would visit us frequently. I remember her face very well and that it was quite white and wrinkled. In her black handbag she always carried little small pieces of licorice. And if we were nice boys she would give us a few little pieces of this licorice, which we all loved. She would, also, give us a piece or so if we just behaved as ordinary children. One day I learned that she passed away, and there was a funeraL We all attended that funeral. It seemed like a pleasant occasion, maybe like some kind of celebration in which everyone dressed up, even the children. Our relatives all came to the funeral, and the relatives I remember the best were my first cousins, from the family of Louis and Annie Mutrux. I must have been around 5-6 years of age, the years being 1921-1922. We children liked each other, and after the funeral we liked enjoyed the fine food that was served. The details of the funeral, the first I had ever attended, are fragmentary: some solemn organ music, a black-garbed minister talking about God and everlasting peace, and a velvety coffin with grandmother inside being lowered into a grave, and some yellow clods of mud escaping from some gray covers around the grave site. I did not understand much about death at that time, maybe that someone was going away for a short trip somewhere. And only in writing these memoirs did I ever pause to think about the impact of my grandmother's death on my mother. She never talked to us about her grief at losing her mother or her father. Now, I wish she had, for it might have given us some idea of how she coped and how we might try to cope with similar events.

At home I can remember, not infrequently, wrestling with my older brother, Edmond. I can remember going to kindergarten at the University City School. It seemed that every day that I went there I got into a fight, and it was usually wrestling with another boy. Usually, I beat up this boy or at least pinned him down. I don't know why I fought so much. It must have been a common thing to do with my brothers. And somebody, either my father or maybe my older brother, Edmond, taught me somewhat how to wrestle and pin somebody down. I was not into hitting another boy, but wrestling seemed quite a fair approach to relating to another boy. And I did so, frequently.

I can visualize the kindergarten at University City School, and I can remember enjoying many of the things we did. The toys, the sandbox and the blocks seemed quite large. I can visualize University City School and kindergarten. I can remember the street, Delmar, and I recall that it took quite a while to get from 7416 Washington, where we lived to the school.

My father sometimes drove us there, maybe that was most of the time, in a Studebaker touring car. It had three rows of seats, and the middle row of seats (jump seats) could be folded. I can visualize it-a bluish color car with a nice loud horn. At school, I rather liked the teacher. I don't recall her name. I liked going to school and doing the things that the kindergarten teacher asked us to do. I remember, also, sometimes going home by streetcar.

There was a place to get that streetcar, probably one end of the line, and there was a Greek restaurant that smelled good. I didn't mind waiting there for the street car. You could get a streetcar that said it went to Clayton and another one that had a label on it that I learned to read and it was Kirkwood-Ferguson. I think I had to take the Clayton car. On that streetcar, I can recall it very well, was a yellowish orange color and it sailed along the tracks. Clickety-clack. It would drop us off somewhere in University City where we would have to wait for a while until one of our parents picked us up. There're some gaps in my memory there of notable events, except for meals and dinners at 7416 Washington. And those were always pleasant memories of eating together in the family.

Then what begins to come back to my mind is the year 1924. I remember that my parents said they were going to Europe. My father, I was told later, had sold a bare lot in St. Louis, and he made some money from that ($10,000 I learned), and he decided that he was going to take the whole family to Europe. But first he was going to go to Provincetown. And he was going to do some painting there, some sketching. And my mother was going to take us four boys across the ocean on a boat and the name of that boat was the President Harding. And we were going to meet papa somewhere in Europe. I will say here that the boat on which we returned from Europe was the Leviathon.

I recall that on the boat we boys had a great time. I understand that we went tourist class, but at that time in my life, I was not aware of any distinctions between accommodations and different classes on these big ships. I did know that there was a certain place on the boat that we boys were not to go; we discovered that and I suppose now that was the first class area where we were not welcome. In any case, I can remember, I must have been around seven years of age, that we boys had a great time on that boat. There were all these ventilators on the decks, we boys loved to climb into these ventilators. Some of them were, possibly, fog horns, I suppose. But we had a great time in climbing into them. There was no sign that said that you couldn't, so when no one was looking, we would climb in. Sometimes I wondered how loud it might be if the boat did get into fog and the foghorns sounded. Later I learned that these vents on the boat were something like horns. They looked something like tubas. They were not all foghorns. Some were ventilators, we discovered, for we could see machinery down into the bowels of the ship. And I have no idea whether or not we could have fallen down them, for obviously we never did. I just remember our getting into them and hanging with our hands on the edge. These were great to hide in. We boys played hide and seek and tag in and around them.

I can recall looking over the edge of the boat, into the ocean. I was aware of the boat rocking, and sometimes we would see fish out in the open ocean. Sometimes we would see the boat discharge rubbish or garbage or papers over the side or the back of the boat. I was not aware at that age that some of these disposal activities might be contaminating the ocean. And I remember that we arrived at Cherbourg. I can vaguely recall seeing the printed name of the town of Cherbourg.

Then we got on a train, which looked different from American trains, and we went to Paris. And let's see. I remember that we then went to a hotel, and mother took us up into our quarters in our hotel room. She asked us to be good boys because she had to go down and do some kind of shopping and had other details to take care of. In any event, we grew somewhat restless in these rooms and decided to play tag and hide and seek. We found a large chiffoniere, discovered that we could open the drawers and Thought wouldn't it be nice and nifty to hide inside the drawers? So we little ones (Charlie and I) climbed inside the drawers and the older ones (Buzzie and Edmond) would close the drawers with us in them. In doing this, something bad happened. The weight of us little boys on the front of the chiffoniere made the whole chiffoniere topple over. It had a large glass mirror, and this large glass mirror broke into many, many pieces. Well, we were rather frustrated regarding what to do. We couldn't hide this whole mess, and we knew mother would be coming back. She did come back and looked it all over. She quickly realized, as we had, that the pieces of glass could not be put together, so she just said calmly that we shouldn't have done that. Then she went downstairs, took us with her to the concierge or to the front desk of the hotel and told the hotel clerk what had happened. Several hotel people went upstairs and looked at the broken chiffonier with this broken glass. They came back downstairs to the hotel lobby and told mother that she would have to pay for the damage. I can visualize her calmly writing out something like a traveler's check and giving it to them. The hotel cleaned up the mess, the broken chiffonier, and replaced it. I cannot remember any time later that our mother reminded us of this catastrophe. She never upbraided us or complained to us about this little event.

From Paris, we went to Lausanne, where some relatives of my mother lived. Their names were Dessuages. There was a very pretty lady; she was a cousin of ours by the name of Marie Louise. There was the mother, whom I can visualize, and a father, a gray-haired man and an elderly woman, but very cheerful, and they did not speak English, only French. Maybe they could also speak German. We spent a fair amount of time with them. Mr. Dessauge, I can recall, often wore a light brown suit and he had white hair and a sporty grayish white mustache. Sometimes he had a cane. I remember that my father, after he had finished his painting in Provincetown, Massachusetts, came and met us. He had a bamboo cane and wore a monocle and spats. (Sometimes, he would let us try on his spats over our shoes, and of course they were huge and looked funny!) We have photographs of him with these spiffy decorations. He was quite a handsome, debonair looking father. We lived in something like an apartment hotel, I suppose, overlooking Lac Leman, and I think you had to walk up many stairs. But there was an elevator, an old fashioned elevator. Well, it probably wasn't old fashioned for those days. I can rather remember the kitchen. And I can remember the bedroom where I stayed with my younger brother, Charlie. I can remember, somehow at that age, making little boats and trains out of matchsticks and paper and gluing them together. I don't know where I got those ideas. But both parents encouraged us to make things, and I appreciate that I can even smell the place now that I think of it. It was a good smell, hard to describe. I can remember playing outside with my brothers, sometime in the morning, and what do you know? Sometimes when it rained, the streets and alleyways would be filled with snails. I thought they looked rather ugly, and when my mother said that sometimes people ate those snails, I couldn't believe it!

One day my younger brother, Charlie, and my older brother, Edmond, were walking down the street towards the little grocery store where I remember the ladies there always said "Bonjour, Madam" and "Merci" to my mother. On the way to that little store where we sometimes bought candy, if we had any money, we saw some kids, around our age. But they were dressed in a comical fashion, in our opinion. There was a boy or girl with long hair and shorts, and I think that one of the kids was wearing some light violet shorts and another smaller child was also wearing shorts. We had on sensible clothes, we thought. They were knickers and long socks and shoes. And these other kids didn't even wear regular shoes. They had on something like sandals. As we passed by, they looked at us and pointed and laughed. And we looked at them and at each other and laughed at them. They said something to us we couldn't understand. And we said something to them in English that they obviously couldn't understand. Pretty soon, we got closer and closer and started making fun of each other. We thought of the worst words that we could and said them to them, and they couldn't understand. And they yelled some harsh words at us. Obviously we couldn't understand what they were saying. We were just about ready to have a fight with them. When my mother came along. And the mother of these kids came out of their house. My mother and their mother began talking with one another. At first they couldn't talk very well because it turned out that these kids were speaking German to us or Swiss-German, and we were speaking English to them. My mother couldn't speak Swiss-German. She knew some German, probably learning it from my father and his parents. Eventually, our mother and their mother found out that they both could speak French. They then began to chat away and speak cordially to one another in a friendly fashion. My mother told us "Well, you can talk to these children. They speak French!" And we did know some French! I may have mentioned that we had learned a French patois growing up in our family, a language that our uncle Louis Mutrux, our mother's brother, always insisted in our speaking to his 12 children during our frequent family visits to his 10-acre farm in St. Louis County. My grandmother was Swiss French and my mother spoke excellent French. We had often been spoken to in French and knew the language. I found it remarkable, even at that age, that when you could speak the same language, kids got along pretty well. Like adults, if they couldn't speak the same language, pretty soon they were ready to get into a fight. Then these mothers came along, found out that they could speak the same language, and we became friends with these kids.

In Lausanne, we learned to roll hoops, up and down the hilly streets, with the Swiss children. That was one of their sports at that time. We also learned to play with their toys: I remember they had some building blocks and railroad trains. We would go down to the lake, Lac Leman, and look along the shore for shells and even fish and go boating. Sometimes we went boating with mother and father. Brother Jules would go along separately in a racing boat, skimming by us rapidly. He was clever!

One of the joys we acquired in Lausanne was eating Swiss chocolate. We especially liked some chocolate candy bars called "Tobleron," triangle-shaped Swiss chocolate with ground nuts. I notice that that brand of candy bar still exists. We had to be nearly perfect to get mother to buy us one of those to divide up amongst ourselves.

We visited various places in Switzerland. Once we visited some relatives living in small Swiss villages. One town was Yverdon. Another, I think, was Orbe. In the latter, we dined with a Swiss family, relatives, and they served us boys some wine and cookies. With just a few sips of wine, I got dizzy. I wondered how the Swiss children at the dining table could tolerate drinking wine. It was hard to understand what mother and father were saying to our Swiss hosts, because they all spoke so rapidly. Sometimes, Mr. Dessauges drove us places in his sporty car, some kind of roadster. We went to the Chateau de Chillion, and we were told gruesome stories about a prisoner who walked around his cell and wore down the stones of his cell. We were also told that some of the prisoners were thrown down holes in the floor and their bodies would be cut up by sharp stationary knives, fixed across the holes, while falling down the hole and before hitting the water of the lake. I, personally, have never got over thinking about and visualizing such a tragic fate.

Mother was always very cheerful and loving in Switzerland. And mother and father seemed very happy with one another. They both went off to visit some relative of my father living in Germany. I think it was in Freiburg, Germany, where my father had a half-brother (Dr. Friedrich Gottschalk) living there who was a physician. The story we were told was that he had been visiting Freiburg before the United States had become engaged in World War 1, and he had not been able to return to the United States. Our parents had left us with a Swiss housekeeper. I can visualize her narrow face and thin body shape. She seemed to be a reasonable child-caretaker to us boys, but she began telling various people in Lausanne, while my parents were in Germany, that she was working for "a nest of German spies." When our parents came back they had to go to the local police station and prove with their passports that we were all American citizens. We kids got questioned by mother about what and how well we were fed. As I reconstruct what might have bothered her, I think she was worrying whether we might have been poisoned. We learned that the housekeeper was mentally ill. These matters did not seem to be of much consequence or danger to us boys, and we soon forgot the episode.

One night, living on about the fifth floor of this apartment building in Lausanne, we heard somebody far away calling for us in English. Somebody in our family, I think it was our mother, finally went downstairs and found that it was our father. He was locked out of the building; apparently the concierge always locked the entrance to the building at night and tenants had to have their own keys to enter. It was papa all right, and he had lost his entrance key. Besides, he was drunk. He explained later to mother and us kids that he had been invited to a bar with Mr. Dessauges and his friends. They all drank copiously. Father told us that the Swiss gentlemen all stuck to drinking Swiss wine and showed off how much they could drink. A competition ensued over who could drink and hold the most liquor, a Swiss or an American. Papa was, certainly, not to be outdone by them, he said. And so he drank not only Swiss wine, but a wide combination of German, French, and British liquors to show these Swiss males that he was a he-man to be recognized seriously. He got very drunk, and belatedly acknowledged (years later) to mother and to us offspring that he had been foolish. But at that time, it was important for a real he-man to show off how much he could drink. In some circle, it is still a way of demonstrating manliness. We never did press father to find out who won the drinking match. Of course, we silently voted and hoped that he did. I don't recall any other time in my life that father became intoxicated with alcohol. It was an episode, however, that we boys -often awed by our very gifted and rather competitive father-remembered, and it helped us realize that the man had some imperfections. But that is another story that doesn't deserve much more attention at this point with the memoirs of our mother.

Well, after a trip up the Alps, from which the views were memorable and which we could see every morning across Lac Leman, we headed back to the United States. We went, this time, on the ocean liner Leviathon, and we boys were told that this was the largest ocean-going passenger ship in service in 1924. It was an adventure again. I can remember scampering around the decks with my brothers. Mother let us run, but she tried to keep an eye on us. Father came up with a phrase he often repeated that we boys were: "touche tous," that is, that we couldn't keep our hands off things and had to touch everything.

I don't know exactly when we boys were told about a change in our parents plans to return to St. Louis, but I suspect that sometime while we were on the Leviathon returning to

New York City or soon thereafter, we were told that we were going to live in New York City for a while. Father, an expert in many things, including musical instruments, got a job selling rare and valuable violins and other string instruments for Wurlitzer. I remember we lived in an apartment overlooking the Hudson River located at 690 Riverside Drive. Our parents explored having us go to private schools, and I remember visiting some. They decided to send us to a public school. Probably it was for financial reasons; I really don't know. The school classes seemed to be fun. But sometimes I would have a belly ache, and mother would write a note to the school which would say, "Louis does not feel well." Mother never questioned my complaints, and I imagine she did the same with my brothers. One day, after losing two front teeth, the school teacher asked me to stand up and recite a lesson. I did so, and after talking for a few minutes some of the other children in the classroom giggled at me. The school teacher, a short nondescript woman, asked me to step out into the school hall with her, and I obediently did so. In an irritated voice, she asked me why I made the school children laugh. I said, pointing to my missing two front teeth, that I had lost my two front teeth, and apologizing I said that I couldn't help lisping a bit. Without hesitation, the teacher slapped me in the face, over my mouth. I whimpered, holding back crying and my tears, and I went back to the classroom with her and sat silently in my chair the rest of the day. I told my mother and father about the episode, and they sympathetically agreed that the teacher should not have slapped me. For a half-dozen times after that episode I would tell mother I had a stomach ache after breakfast in the morning, and she would say that I didn't have to go to school that morning. She would write her little notes for me saying: "Louis does not feel well."

Nothing much was said in our family about this event. I don't think my mother or father complained to the school about it. And I forgot about it. All I noticed was that I was afraid to get up and recite at school, although I very much wanted to do so. I had to force myself to do so. To get over this, I often voluntecred to recite or to be in plays. Not for many years later, during my training psychoanalysis in Chicago while I was learning to become a psychoanalyst, did I recognize that this event at school produced a mild school phobia in me that I dealt with by "overcompensation," forcing myself to perform, although unaccountably anxious about performing. At the time of my personal psychoanalysis, I was 32 years of age, and I didn't experience much "stage fright" with verbal performances-only slight "stage fright".

Mother was always around, helping us here and everywhere, in New York City. Father was away at work, selling fine violins and so forth. We boys must have tested the limits of parental endurance. We were allowed freedom to go and come as we desired. There was a dumb-waiter in our apartment. And, of course, we boys bad to try it out, get into it, and go to the floor below and above us. Our mother didn't want us to do that we found out. So we were good boys, and we stopped this pleasure. We were allowed to go down to the Hudson River bank and play. We had to cross some railroad tracks. We recognized that most of the trains were switch engines, moving around passenger and freight cars. The men involved with the trains didn't seem to mind some little boys crossing their tracks to get to the river. On the river, we played boats, that is, we made little paper or wood boats and put them in the river and watched them move away. One time, on the river bank we found a large door with some tarpaper nailed onto it. We got the good idea that this would make a good raft. And like Huckleberry Finn, we could go out on the raft in the river and have fun. Somehow I was the one kid that decided to get on the raft, after we had successfully dragged it into the water. The raft wasn't big enough to hold me up high out of the water, so I took my shoes and socks off and let my feet get wet. It was fun. I had a short pole and pushed out into the current. Then the pole became too short to use. It didn't touch bottom any more, and the current caught me. I drifted more than 50 feet from the shore. My brothers hollered for me to swim back to shore, but I couldn't really swim that well. I was only seven. In this dilemma, my brothers got a good idea They went up to the railroad tracks, stopped one of the switch engines, and asked the engineers to help them help me get back to shore. These were good men. One of them came to the shore with a rope and he was going to lasso me and bring me to the shore. I didn't like that idea and, furthermore, he couldn't pitch the rope as far out as I was. I don't know how they managed, but the railroad workers phoned somebody, and a man came out in a boat and took me ashore. I was pretty cold by that time, about 200 feet from shore and drifting away. And I must admit, I was scared. The railroad workers told us to be careful next time and not try rafting. But they didn't say we couldn't come down to the river side. I remember other times playing on an anchored replica of the ship known as the DeWitt Clinton that had been used in some movie. We played on board several times. We would tell mother about our adventures, and she might say to be careful. But she never dissuaded us from being little explorers. New York City and the particular vicinity where we lived was apparently fairly safe for young boys at that time. We enjoyed our life there. And then, after being there for one year, our parents told us that we were returning to St. Louis, Missouri.

We returned to St Louis, and instead of moving into our home on 7416 Washington in University City, Missouri, where my parents had rented it to Professor David Barr, MD., Chairman of the Department of Internal Medicine, Washington University School of Medicine, we moved to an apartment at 6000 Waterman Avenue in St. Louis, a six-family apartment building that my parents owned. This apartment building had been built by my namesake uncle Louis Mutrux. Part of the building was built on an old bridge pier that had held a bridge over the Des Peres river. There were only three bedrooms in this apartment, and for six people that was fairly crowded. But we boys did not realize it was crowded, for we thought that was just the way living arrangements were supposed to be. My father had a room for himself.

Mother sometimes slept in a bedroom where Edmond and I slept. Sometimes she slept on a sofa in the dining room. I think brother Jules and Charles slept together in a room on a back porch. My brother Charles and I attended Hamilton Elementary School, and I believe brother Edmond went to Ben Blewett Junior High School, and brother Jules went to Soldan High School. There were two wooden garages behind the apartment, where we stored many things, and sometimes the family automobile would go into one of those garages. Since my parents owned this apartment, we were allowed to spread out into the basement and, eventually, take over a room that had originally been intended for the janitor, a black gentleman by the name of William Pruitt. Father built a little house in the back yard for us boys; he was rather handy at building houses. Besides being a violin and piano virtuoso, composer, fine artist, and writer and music and art critic for the St. Louis Post Dispatch, he was a very good whittler. I know about the latter, because he whittled a saber, straight sword, and small dagger for three of us boys out of white pine. Father and mother did not discourage us–in but fact encouraged us three younger brothers to each build a "clubhouse" on the banks of the Des Peres river. Where did we get the building materials? We got them from the discarded wood piles, and sometimes from the undiscarded wood, at new construction in our nearby neighborhood. My house was a narrow one with a peaked roof and a single narrow door in front The best "clubhouse" (next to the one father built that had windows with real glass panes in it) was the one Edmond built. It had a "spy tower," about 15 feet high I estimate. And it had a tunnel on the floor of it that ended up a few yards outside of his "clubhouse's boundaries." Charlie's house was just a plain squarish house with a flat roof.

Mother would make sandwiches for us, and we could go and eat them in our separate houses or have a party in one of them. We acquired a lot of local boyfriends around our ages. They were always welcome to help us make our houses and play in them. I don't remember how it came about, but we three boys got the idea of digging a network of tunnels along the Des Péres riverbanks, and we made it stretch out, like a maze, for about 75 or more feet. The tunnels were covered with boards and dirt, and they were, therefore, well hidden. To crawl somewhere in the tunnels, you needed a candle or flashlight. With a few chosen friends we could have secret meetings. I don't recall that Jules got involved in building a "clubhouse" or tunnels. He was, of course, older than we were. And he had more grown-up endeavors. I remember he got into making bows and arrows. And he became an expert at making big bows out of hickory or lemon wood. We younger brothers looked up to him as somewhat of a marvel in making such things, and he was a nice enough big brother to show us younger ones how to shoot arrows with them. I remember he taught me how to use them. Then, he got interested in radios and amplifiers, and he built a big one in the apartment house basement. Of course, he had to test how loudly it could be made to play; mother had to tell him not to play it so loudly, because the apartment tenants were complaining. Then Jules got interested in automobiles, and I recall he had a friend who owned a Stanley Steamer, and this friend would sometimes bring it and park it in front of our apartment building. We boys looked at it in wonder and fascination. Jules was not to be outdone by his friend's Stanley Steamer. He bought a Mercer, and told us that it was the fastest auto around and that it had an all aluminum engine. He took me for a ride once, and it was scary because he drove so fast, it also bothered me that one of the tires was held onto the tire rim with a couple of ropés. I never did understand that mechanical arrangement.

Jules liked to speed. I remember mother telling him not to drive so fast. We had a number of family cars. Father liked cars. We had a Studebaker, then a Whippet, then a Moon, and so on. Then Edmond got old enough and got money to buy a car. He got an old model T Ford roadster (for $25). If I was good, he would let me borrow it. He later got a model A Ford. (I think papa helped him buy it if he would stop smoking cigarettes. He did stop for a while.)

I notice I seem to be temporarily leaving out mother in this narrative. The marvelous thing about her was that she maintained a high interest in the activities of each one of us boys. I didn't notice that she had any favorites. I will admit that when I was younger, I observed that she was fussing over my little brother Charlie and telling him what a fine looking and good boy he was. I thought he was fine looking too and that he was okay. But I recall asking mother (We somehow most often called her by her first name, Kelmie, or shortened it to "me"), "What's wrong "me," don't I have my dimple any more?" She assured me that my dimple was still there.

I should not overlook father's role in our child rearing, although these memoirs are purposely focused on mother. Father liked to go out sketching in public parks and in rural areas. I think he would go quite often, maybe as much as twice a week. And often he would invite us boys and one or two of our friends. Some favorite places for us were Forest Park and Rock Hill Creek and Quarry. At the latter place, we could go swimming in the creek and explore the neighboring woods. We tried swimming in the water ways (lakes and streams) in Forest Park, but the Park Police did not always approve of our swimming there, especially when we were in the nude. During the hot summers in St. Louis it was very tempting to go in those cool waters. Our father did not encourage us to break the rules of the Park Police, if there were such rules. But one time, on a very very hot summer day, about 8-10 of us boys went swimming under a park bridge to cool off. It was delightful! But the Park Police discovered us. And they made us all march out from under the bridge and lined us up on the public asphalt road over the bridge, out in public view of all autos passing by. They lectured us, and we pleaded innocent, lying a bit and saying that we didn't know there was any such rule about no swimming, and besides, we didn't see any sign saying "NO SWIMMING." The policemen, there were three, talked together, saying aloud that maybe they should take us to jail, which worried us greatly. Then they took a second look at brother Edmond and noticed, in his nudity, that he was the only boy who had sprouts of pubic hair. They gathered around him, and asked how old he was and that he should know better. The police asked each other aloud whether they should take only Edmond to jail. Then, acting quite forgiving and big-hearted, they said that they would let us go this time, but if they caught us swimming another time we knew what would happen.

When we got home, one of us told mother what had happened. She was naturally concerned. She arranged for us to go swimming on hot summer days at the Coliseum, a large public swimming pool in downtown St. Louis that admitted swimmers at a low cost (I think) or at another smaller public swimming pool. Whenever it could be arranged, she also took us out to St. Louis County where our uncle Louis lived and had 10 acres of farmland and a swimming pool that he and his sons had built. Boy, that was really a treat! For we not only loved swimming there, but we adored our first cousins. (As I mentioned before there were 12 of them.)

I don't know how mother got the ideas, but she arranged for us to go other places. We used to go out to Creve Coeur, a rural amusement park with all kinds of rides and water pleasures. The ride out to that amusement park was, itself, a ball. The ride took place in open street cars, often several hitched together, that sped along into and through forested places. She also took us out to a place called "Cottage Farms," along a small river, and where we would stay overnight. There was music and dancing at night. I wanted to be able to dance with the young folks, but my brother Charlie and I were too young. Besides, we didn't know how to dance with a partner, and we couldn't figure out very well how the dancers were able to avoid stepping on each others' feet or even keep together. That was a mystery we would have to grow up more to learn about. Mother seemed to enjoy these outings to Cottage Farm and other such places as much as we did. Usually, somehow, father didn't come along on most of these outings.

I think mother met someone at Cottage Farm who told her that a good experience for us kids would be to spend a week on a farm with some real farmers. Mother arranged this. And we saw how a busy farm family cultivated their crops, fed their livestock, milked their cows, and kept house. Edmond, Charlie, and I stayed at this farm family's house. It was very plain and natural. I remember one of the sons driving us in a truck to the small neighboring town, about 3-4 miles from their home. We shopped with them at the County Store and went to the Post Office. The oldest son taught us to ride a mule. The mule seemed very large to me and, surprising, gentle. He asked me one day whether I would like to ride the mule to the little town to the Post Office, mail some letters, and get the mail. I said sure. He showed me how to steer the mule. It seemed a huge animal to sit on and amazingly obedient to be guided by a little boy. So off I went, headed for the Post Office. I felt very confident and grown up, riding that large animal on a dirt road, far out in the country, with no other people in sight, I imagined myself like a country gentleman riding his horse, something that I might have seen in the moving pictures. The mule ambled along and at a certain point, I don't know why, it stopped. I was riding bare back. I said "giddap" and when there was no forward movement, I said all the other words I could think of; and there was no progress. Then I dug my heels into the animal's side, and I was encouraged because the mule began to amble forward again. This stopping of the mule and starting happened three or four more times before I got to my destination. I tried to think what the mule was thinking that made it pause and stop. Was it lazy, stubborn, unwilling, trying to show who was the boss? I thought maybe all these ideas applied to what the mule was thinking. After delivering and getting new mail to take home, I figured the mule would probably know it was heading home and would walk and, even, run a bit. Not so. It still stopped and paused occasionally, a few times to munch on some grass by the roadside. At other times, it just stopped and looked around. I tried talking to it and digging my heels into its flank The results were never immediate. The mule must have decided that I was a different human being than it was used to, and that I was not much to be afraid of, and that it could move along at any pace it wanted to. It mostly did so, being barely influenced by my efforts to keep it moving. Still, for a little boy, the experience the mule gave me taught me first-hand about what the word "mulish" means.

The experience at Cottage Farm and with rural Missouri farm life blends in with other events orchestrated and managed by my mother. She unobtrusively arranged to help each different son carry out his diverse activities and roles that were ordained by his differences, inheritance, temperament, innate skills, personality, and personal preferences. She was always there, available, personally interested, enthusiastic and concerned about each son's individuality, aspirations, performance, and activities.

Of course, for my mother there were the normally expected requirements of married life and attending to the requirements of our father. We boys did not at all realize that mother was a gourmet cook, without appearing to try to be. Her cooking was influenced, now I realize, by her Swiss-French heritage. Oh yes, there were the fine feasts we enjoyed when the family finances were good. Roast lamb, leg of lamb, roast beef, roast pork, chicken, kidneys, kidney stew, vegetables of all kinds. And great desserts. Somehow I became a picky eater, and there were certain vegetables I didn't want to eat, like spinach, tomatoes, turnips, and squash. I didn't know why at the time. They didn't taste good to me. Now on reflection, I believe that finicky eating followed some episodes of some sicknesses during which I vomited, and the color, texture, and ingredients of my vomitus reminded me of some of those foods. Anyway, many years later I overcame my dislile of these foods. But during my period of finicky eating, mother would encourage me to try to eat these foods, but she would never force me. We did sometimes hear her say to us, however, when we left food on our plates, "Remember the starving Armenians." I vaguely remember her explaining to us who the "starving Armenians" were, and how they happened to be starving after we repeatedly asked who they were. I think my rather poor eating habits started shortly after the age of 6 when I was taken to the hospital (Aeolian Brothers Hospital) to have a tonsillectomy and adenoidectomy and, of all things, a circumcision (for "phimosis"). Our family doctor (Dr. Leon) said he thought I should have such operations, the doctor at the Hospital agreed, and that's what was done. Mother took me to the Hospital, and the nurses were so friendly and warm that I thought maybe I was going to some kind of party where grown-ups wore white uniforms. I can remember the smell of the hospital, something like a disinfectant. I slept overnight there, and I felt a little lonesome for home. The friendly nursing staff came and got me, put me on a stretcher, and wheeled me into an operating room. That seemed rather fun but unnecessary, for I could easily have walked. Then they sort of lifted little me to what I realize now was an operating table. Besides the operating table, which had a big light over it, was a tray with an assembly of tools on it; I had never seen instruments like these. They mostly seemed to have sharp edges on them. Soon a doctor and a nurse came in. One of them said that I was going to be given something to smell and that it didn't smell good or bad and that it would put me to sleep. I know now that I was given ether to smell. It didn't smell very good, and it put me to sleep fast. I woke up later and I had a sore throat, and I had a bandage on the end of my penis. When I swallowed it hurt. When I tried to urinate it burned badly. I was shocked at the cruelty of these people who were in the medical profession. As if to make amends, my parents came in to visit me and brought me ice cream. I tasted the ice cream, and on swallowing it my throat complained loudly. Now I was silently angry with my parents, whom I figured were part of what I experienced as a conspiracy.

I go back in time a bit to tell this little side story to report that mother was obviously very concerned and troubled with my convalescence. I didn't want to eat very much, and I lost weight. I walked around in a pitiful way, hunched up, looking dreary, and sort of cupping my hands over my genital area. My mother conferred with her loving sister-in-law, Aunt Annie, who lived way out in St Louis County and had twelve children of her own. It was now summer time, and the weather was hot in St Louis. These two allies, mother and aunt Annie, decided that little Louis might be helped if he joined the Mutrux children, all twelve of them, and went out to live on uncle Louis' farm for a while. The Mutrux children were cordial. We had to speak French to one another, unless we privately talked in English when uncle Louis was out of earshot. I slept in a bed on the porch of their house with three other children. Running around the farm, looking at the chickens pecking away at their food, helping collect eggs, watching the cow get milked by one of the Mutrux boys, and swimming with my cousins in the pool that uncle Louis made did, somehow, have curative effects on my ailments. I did get rehabilitated, and my sore places healed. The sore body parts worked well again. I still feel indebted to aunt Annie Mutrux and my cousins for helping me overcome, at least superficially, the aftermath of these operations. Somehow I feel surgery on children should be sparing and as infrequent as possible.

The family trip to Europe, specifically, France and Switzerland, took place the next year when I was 7. I forgot all about the surgery I underwent, I thought, and I greatly enjoyed life in Switzerland. I should add that my personal psychoanalysis did dredge up feelings of human betrayal and memories of emotional and physical pains suffered during my tonsillectomy, adenoidectomy, and circumcision that have helped me to be especially sympathetic and empathetic to children and adults who have undergone surgery.

Now, after this flashback, which grew from reminiscences over my dear mother's good cooking and how it was that I became a finicky eater for a while, let us touch on how this mother of ours functioned as a cuisiniere during the years of the so-called Great Depression, beginning in 1929. Mother managed to feed four hungry boys by feeding us soups, stews, fresh bread, and cakes, like gingerbread, lemon cake, angel cake, chocolate cake, and so forth that she made in a large cake pan. She managed to feed all of us on $1.00 per day. That was 6 people! Of course, the dollar was worth a lot more then than it is now. During those days of the Depression, we all seemed to have hearty appetites. No food was left on our plates.

Growing up in West St Louis, Missouri, was fun. Forest Park was nearby, and we often went there. We went hiking to the Jefferson Memorial, a left-over from the 1904 World's Fair, a repository of collectors' items from that the Civil War and later. We frequently went to the St. Louis Art Museum. There they seemed to like children, and we were invited to participate in lectures on art and drawing contests. If we did well in the drawing, we might be rewarded with a postcard of a famous work of art in the Museum. Sometimes we stayed overnight in Forest Park, which was safe in those days, and we were allowed to do so. Sometimes we looked for golf balls in the rough of the St. Louis Municipal Golf Course, and if we found some, we discovered we could get as much as 25 cents for a good one. We also looked in the water holes for golf balls, and we discovered if we went wading in them, we could find some, feeling them under our feet in the muddy bottom. It was like discovering Easter eggs, worth money!

We three younger boys were very explorative. We would go into new apartments or residences being built near where we lived. If the workmen were not around, we would climb the scaffolding and see how high we could go. It's a wonder we didn't fall and hurt ourselves, but we were lucky and only suffered minor hurts. I remember that we discovered we could climb up and down large chimneys, by pressing our knees out against one side and our back against the other side. Once I was half way down a brick chimney , and one of the kids at the top accidentally knocked a loose brick off the top, which hit me on the head. I yelped and cried. The brick drew some blood, but the cut stopped bleeding. I crawled out of the partially built chimney, and complained to whomever knocked the brick onto me, not to do such a careless thing again. Ah, now that I think of it, the result could have been much worse! Ignorance sometimes helps.

In those days, papa wasn't able to get very many jobs as a musician. He composed classical music, which didn't sell. He worked and headed a string quartet that once in a long while got a commission to play. He sold fine art at Newhouse galleries, he sold his own paintings (landscapes and portraits), he sold vacuum cleaners, he gave music lessons, privately, or for the Hugo School of Music. From my viewpoint as a young son, it seemed to me that he took the financial depression more as a challenge than as an overwhelming defeat. On the other hand, I came to know how perfectionistic and exacting he was as a music teacher or as the leader of his own string quartet. I knew he aspired to a high level of greatness as a musician, composer, and artists. And here, at times, he was teaching little children how to play not just the violin or piano but, of all instruments, the accordion. And I knew, from personal experience, he was not always a patient gentleman. Anyway, I didn't hear him complain of the burdensome aspects of earning a livelihood for a family. He seemed to accept that this was his job description and being a breadwinner was automatically his responsibility without question. We children were expected to earn whatever monies we could at a fairly young age. We were allowed to keep and spend the money we earned ourselves. Mother, especially, encouraged us to save our bits of change and got us small banks in which to put our pennies, nickels, and dimes. Our parents owned the apartment house in which we lived. It was a six-family apartment structure. We children were given the privilege of making money by helping decorate the apartments for old or new tenants. We might get $1.00 for painting a whole kitchen, later up to $2.00, which included painting the ceiling and walls. Those amounts of money were good in the 1920's and 1930's. The paints were all oil paints, not the water-based paints available today. We might get $.50 to $1.00 varnishing the floor of one room. For some reason, I didn't like to varnish floors. I preferred to put shellac on them. I think that was so because the shellac dried so fast and varnish did not

In my teens, I learned the value of a dollar and the cost of taking out a girl. If I shoveled into the basement the soft coal, say 5 tons of coal, I would get $.50 per ton. Ten tons of coal would net me $5.00, which would allow me to take out a date in my teens, buy gasoline for the family car, buy a meal and drinks for the girl, and take her to a school dance. All the hours and energy it took to shovel the coal into a wheelbarrow, roll the wheelbarrow to an opening in the basement, and dump the coal down the coal chute helped me realize the cost of dating and mating. If I didn't want to do the job, my brother Edmond would do it. I don't remember whether Charlie did such a job, but I suspect he did so or something equivalent to it to earn money and his way in life. Anyway, the cost of taking out a girl didn't deter me from taking her out because I really liked girls. And I didn't stick to one girl at that time, but I dated many different ones.

As I have already said, it was mother who looked into what jobs should be done at the six family apartment house where we lived and which we owned. A new tenant or an old tenant might require some improvement or decorating in their apartment. Mother would decide what should be done, and then she would negotiate with one of us boys concerning what would be done and who would do it for what price. I can remember a few times telling her I didn't want to do the job at the price she offered, complaining it was too much work She would usually go along with our request, and most of the time the financial reward she offered was acceptable.

Father was rarely involved in these kinds of decisions. He earned money for the family through his music or art. For a while, he played violin in the St. Louis Symphony orchestra. Sometimes he played the piano or violin in movie houses during the silent film era. He organized several different string quartets, and he managed to obtain money from well-to-do people to support the string quartet. Father would get a commission to paint someone's portrait or to do a landscape. Sometimes, he bought and sold string instruments and made some money that way. He also gave music lessons, privately or through the Hugo School of Music.

Mother, on the other hand, handled most of the business matters involving the real estate our parents owned. These amounted to the apartment house in which we lived and partial ownership, with uncle Louis Mutrux, of an apartment house in Clayton, Missouri, a suburb of St. Louis. We boys were involved through mother's interventions in trying to keep the apartment house where we lived in satisfactory condition in order to rent our apartments. Through the depression years, beginning in 1929, the apartment house on 6000 Waterman Avenue kept us going financially, for father's jobs were few during those years.

Often we might try bargaining with mother about what we might be paid for a job, like painting the kitchen, varnishing or shellacking a floor, painting the woodwork in one of the bedrooms. We became experts in repairing the roof, and we were proud to be able to climb up on the roof of this three-story apartment and see the view around us and below us from this vantage point. In writing these memoirs now, I can begin to understand how we became expert do-it-yourselfers. And many years later, each one of us boys was rather skilled at fixing and keeping our home in good repair. I often wondered why some male contemporaries of mine were unable to repair and fix things around their home. Obviously, they were never expected to learn these skills as children. When I later bought a run-down 180 acre farm in Indiana–about 50 miles from Cincinnati where I was living and lived there from 1955 to

1967– I did a lot of rebuilding and repairing of the house and barns there, some with the help of my brother, Edmond, and my wife, Helen, and my son, Guy. Somehow I really enjoyed doing these things, in part because these activities were so different from my rather sedentary life as a neuropsychiatrist and psychoanalyst in the Department of Psychiatry at the University of Cincinnati. The other reasons for enjoying doing these repairing and building activities included the sheer pleasure of making and creating things. I certainly was not a fancy carpenter or repair man. I was fairly competent, as were my older brothers and father, after whom I followed along. Mother encouraged us boys to do these things, and her monetary rewards for our work helped reinforce the idea in our heads that our capacity to learn how to do these jobs was good and worthwhile. Our first cousins, the Mutrux children, were brought up by their parents to do the same sort of constructive activities.

The years of our living at 6000 Waterman Avenue in St. Louis, Missouri extended, for me, from second grade elementary school at Hamilton School, through Ben Biewett Junior High, Soldan High, Hadley Vocational School, Washington University night school while I worked as a bank clerk at the first National Bank (from 1935-1936), Washington University day school (1936-1940), Washington University Medical School (1940-December, 1943), medical internship at Barnes Hospital, and neuropsychiatric residency (1943-1946). Mother was available, more than father, to occasionally help us with our homework and participate in the local Parent Teachers Association. As I remember it, she was equally interested in the academic progress of each of her boys. She nurtured the gifts and skills of each boy, letting his natural inclinations determine his directions. We certainly seemed different from each other in our personalities and academic inclinations. But there is no question that we were surrounded by, if not immersed, in a musical, artistic, and literary milieu, influenced by father and his friends, mother, uncle Louis and aunt Annie Mutrux and their big family, which eventually became 12 children. Some of the tenants of our apartment house contributed to this milieu, especially Frank Martindale Webster and Henry Thoma, both professors of English at Washington University, who took an interest especially in my older brother, Max Jules, and in me. In my years of attending Washington University-after my older brother, Jules, had majored there in Art History and my brother Edmond had studied Fine Arts there–Frank Webster encouraged me to read systematically many of the books in his extensive collection and listen to symphonic music while following the scores. But those details are getting ahead of my unfolding narrative.

There we lived at 6000 Waterman, in a lower to middle-class neighborhood, with Catholic, Protestant, and Jewish friends–all Caucasian. I can remember many of the names of the kids we played with. Robert Meyer: We used to play corkball in his back yard, and I got pretty good at it. I heard that this ball game was invented in St. Louis. Wilbur Dillon: He was head of the Dillon gang, a bunch of boys who lived a couple blocks away. We used to fight them. We threw rocks at each other, and I never knew why. We later all made friends with them because most of us became members of the same Boy Scout troop. Ed and Richard Torlina: They were nice boys. The younger brother, Richard, died from kidney disease when he was in his early twenties. I had lost track of him, but when I was a young doctor and intern in medicine at Barnes Hospital in St Louis, I was rather shocked to learn that the diseased kidneys I was shown at Pathology Rounds belonged to Richard Torlina! I reflected then that I was in a strange profession that might expose me to other similar personal experiences that I would find unpleasant. Jack Nader: He said I wouldn't go to heaven because I wasn't Catholic. He was a good fighter. Our older friends put boxing gloves on both of us and urged us to fight. I did not particularly want to fight him, for I had nothing about which to get into a fight with him. But the older kids explained that boxing was a sport, and it was okay to see who was better at it. During the boxing match he hit me in the nose, and it bled. The older boys stopped the fight We still were friends, but I never forgot that he had a strong right hand punch and that I needed to learn to guard my nose. Because of that experience, I found I preferred to wrestle rather than box if I was put into a situation where I was expected to fight another boy. Some years later, I remember he broke his leg, and I visited him at his home to comfort him because it was not healing very well. Also, there was Jack Miravelle: He grew to be a big fellow, and he played football at college. When he was still a young boy, he showed us how to masturbate. And there was Eric Smith: A next door neighbor, who grew up to be a famous St. Louis architect. We played together with toys and games at his house. I don't remember why we one day had a wrestling match. I pinned him.

We used to play football during our high school years with these friends. It was tackle-football rather than touch football, and none of us wore protective uniforms or helmets. It's a wonder we didn't get badly injured. I think playing that type of football, "sandlot" football, was how Jack Nader broke his leg. A little way down the street from us, on Waterman Avenue, lived Helen Krummenacher. She was a beauty! For quite a while she was one of my girl friends. She was quite popular! Her father was a pharmacist, and he had a big drug store at Kingshighway and Delmar. He employed me during some summers in swell jobs, like running the soda fountain or working behind the cigarette and cigar counter. Making sodas and ice creams sundaes was fun, and I served mostly kids and young people. Working behind the cigarette and cigar counter was quite a different experience. It was a very busy place to work. Besides all the different kinds of smokes, there were snuffs and chewing tobaccos that I had to learn about. I can recall feeling hurried to make change for customers, who often waited in line for service. I think mother and father were pleased that I had such a job. Mother encouraged me to try to save some money. Many years later, I learned that the Swiss people have a reputation for being frugal, and I guess I was being gently programmed by mother to follow the Swiss teaching.

I wonder what ever happened to all those friends?

I got a job. That was after graduating from Soldan High School in December 1933 and going to Hadley Vocational School from January 1934 to December 1934. My job was at the First National Bank in St. Louis. And I rather lost track of all those elementary and high school friends. Disappointed at not being able to go to Washington University, where my two older brothers had gone or were going, because of the "Great Depression," while working during the day at the First National Bank as a courier for stocks and bonds, then as a personnel clerk, and finally in the transit department, I went to Washington University Night School four nights a week to learn what College was like. I was, of cause, encouraged to do so by both my father and mother. I did well academically. In fact, on the basis I guess of my night school grades, I was able to get a half-scholarship, which enabled me to start full-time at Washington University, beginning in September 1936. Mother gave me moral support. And so did father. But they could not help me very much in the financial area. Actually, I was able to get jobs at the University. There were federally funded jobs that paid $.45/hour if you worked on the campus and jobs that paid $.60/hour if you worked off the campus. And also, I did some tutoring. I spent part of my second year at Washington University, one or two evenings a week, helping a wealthy Country Day School, a private school, student, John Funsten, learn how to study and prepare for examinations. I performed like a caring older brother with him, and he learned how to become a good student. I found I enjoyed his company, my teaching relationship with him, and the financial compensation I earned. No doubt experiences of this sort contributed to my deciding to become an academician later. And furthermore, such experiences contributed to my aspiring to become a physician and psychiatrist.

During my four years at Washington University, my parents were always emotionally supportive. I loved going to the University. I liked the subject matter of every course I took. I did not like the pressure put on me by the Organic Chemistry course I took, for the Professor warned us that he might spring examinations on us. And he frequently did so. But all of us in this Organic Chemistry course were in the same boat and were forced to make studying this subject high priority.

I found extra-curricular activities at Washington University fascinating. I liked being in plays, writing for the College newspaper (Student Life) or magazine (The Eliot), being active in minor sports, like fencing and swimming. The social life was truly fun and helped me learn a great deal about interpersonal relations.

Of course, I could not afford to join a social fraternity. There is an amusing story about that. During the summer of 1936, while waiting to matriculate at Washington University, I had a phone call from a young man, asking me whether he could visit me at home. I said sure. Along came two young men, and they asked me to join them at their fraternity house, which was fairly close to where I lived. I went there, and a group of young men talked to me and asked me about my scholastic and career goals. I chattered away about them. Several of them asked to be excused to talk in another room for a few minutes, and then they returned. They jointly talked about their all being members of a social fraternity (I don't remember the name) and then they asked me whether I wanted to join theirs. I told them that my financial resources were very limited and that I did not believe I could afford to do so. Well, they said they could make some kind of adjustment for me so that I could do so. They explained that they were one of the first Jewish fraternities to appear on the campus of Washington University. I was slightly embarrassed about this situation. But I went ahead and told them that I had a feeling that I might not really be acceptable to them. How could that be, they inquired almost in unison? Well, I fumbled, I am not Jewish. I go to the Grace Methodist Episcopal church at Skinker and Waterman , and my religious heritage is Protestant and Catholic. The faces of several of the fraternity brothers reddened. And several asked to go to the adjoining room for a moment. They soon returned. And one of the fraternity brothers told me, with a very serious expression, that I could not become a member of their fraternity since I was not Jewish. We all shook hands. And I left. I told my parents about this episode, and they both chuckled.

Along this line, I was classified as an Independent on the Washington University campus. Since I was very active in extra-curricular affairs, I had lots of acquaintances, not only among the other independents, but among the fraternities and sororities. Father told me that at the University of Missouri at Columbia, Missouri, he was quite active as a Sigma Nu, and he enjoyed his fraternity life. Once in a while he talked about certain Sigma Nu fraternity brothers with whom he spoke and/or corresponded. Beginning the second year of my attending Washington University, I began to be invited by girls to take them to their sorority dances, which I really enjoyed. I was a good dancer, and I was fairly good looking and easy to meet. So that may explain why girls liked to invite me to take them to their sorority Prom. Also, I had some good friends who were fraternity members, especially among the Sigma

Alpha Episilons (SAE's). A number of them edited or wrote for the Washington U. newspaper (Student Life) and magazine (Eliot), and I became friends with them because I often wrote for both these publications. They were particularly cordial and often invited me to visit their fraternity house on the Washington University campus. Neither mother nor father made any memorable comments about my social life when I was a University student , except to remark that I seemed to be rather popular. I think mother was equally preoccupied with my three brothers, my father's activities and life, her own responsibilities with family financial affairs, and her own rather active social life with nearby relatives (the Mutrux family, the Nott family, and others), and the Alliance Francaise. Oh yes, she loved that organization, and once in a while she encouraged me to attend and even meet some French-speaking girls my age. Mother was also involved with friends of relatives. There was the Knudsen family, who had about 13-14 children and were friends of and belonged to the same church as the Mutrux family. The father and uncle Knudsen were both string instrument musicians who played in father's string quartet, and we would often hear the quartet playing and father scolding or advising how some quartet should be played. Mother was, come to think of it, a very social person just with friends and neighbors. But mother would never miss coming to a play, musical comedy, graduation exercise or any other University event in which I was involved. I don't know why, but father rarely, if ever, showed up at these events. I never felt slighted by him over his absence. I just figured he was busy, somewhere, trying to earn a living, and he and mother had a fair division of labor with respect to their child care-taking. Mother would also come to gatherings at the Grace Methodist Episcopal Church, where Edmond, Charlie, and I went to Vacation Bible School. Later we were active in the Boy Scouts. At the Grace Methodist Episcopal Church I sang in the Church Choir, a group of about 75 people, which sang regularly on the radio. I got free singing lessons. I know I was rather mediocre as a singer, but I enjoyed the church music, and I did not sing very loudly. I acted in a few religious plays at church. Mother and father did not attend this Church, In fact, they did not go to Church. Mother encouraged us to attend, though, and she usually gave us a little money to put in the offering plate. She always made our apartment available for any church related activities, like the High-League, Cub Scout Meetings. I became a Cub Scout Leader, somehow, probably because as a well-behaved Boy Scout I was invited to be a leader of younger boys who were Cub Scouts. Because I achieved the standing of a Life Scout—I faltered in the process of working to become an Eagle Scout--the scoutmaster appointed me to be Patrol Leader of the Horse PatroL Ha ha, I laugh softly now when I think of the name of the Patrol, and how seriously I took my responsibility. I can remember the scoutmaster, Mr. Robinson, he was both serious and sincere. And mother, she always facilitated our going to Camp-Outs or Boy Scout Camp or the YMCA Camp. We were aware that money was sometimes scarce, but she always seemed to scrape together enough money to send us to these camps. Now I wonder how she got the idea to do so in the first place. I know that these camping experiences were good for me. I learned how to be "a good camper" and get along with large groups of other boys besides my brothers. Later I was able to get a paying job as a Camp Counsellor at a well-to-do Boys Camp, Camp Nebagamon, in Wisconsin. My earnings at that camp helped pay some of my tuition expenses at Washington University School of Medicine, where I later went from September 1940 through December 1943. But that is a story that I will talk about more later.

During the last two years of my University life, 1939-1940, I pondered what I wanted to do career-wise. I had taken extra course work during these academic years, for I seemed to have boundless energy and enthusiasm to learn. So I had majors in English, Psychology, and Biology. I had, also, taken all the required premedical courses, because I had become interested in the idea of becoming a psychiatrist, though there was no likelihood of my having the financial means to attend medical school. If Washington University had had a strong clinical psychology graduate school I would have probably attended it, but at that time Washington University had an outstanding Department of Psychophysiology and Experimental Psychology. Only a few undergraduate courses in normal and abnormal psychology were available. I learned that to become a clinician of abnormal psychology I would have to go to medical school, which would be one of the stepping stones to becoming a psychiatrist or neuropsychiatrist. In any event, here I was as a college student, enjoying all the variety of courses I took, aiming loosely to pursue psychology, biology, a writing career, possibly a legal career, maybe an academic career. I was an honor student with a very high grade-point average. Surprisingly my father, who had always preached to us boys to seek a career which we loved (a guiding principle that led him not to practice law as his father had, but to become a journalist, composer, musician, and artist), suddenly advised me not to consider going to post-graduate school in medicine or psychology, but to become a business man. I had become bold enough to remind him how he had preached to us sons to follow our own inclinations. And he retorted he had changed his mind with respect to my situation. "The United States of America is a land of business men. You did well at the First National Bank of St. Louis. Why don't you stick to what you do well in?" he said. I told him that I did fairly well in other subjects, too, and I would like to be able to go to medical school. He scratched his head in wonderment, musing that his half-brother, Friedrich, had become a doctor. But he wondered aloud whether I had been influenced by Professor Frank Webster to aspire to become a neuropsychiatrist. I suppose he might have been a touch jealous that Frank Webster was among my mentors. But Frank Webster never did suggest to me what I should aim to become career-wise.

Anyway, the summer of 1939, I had a job at St. Albans, Missouri, the 10,000 acre estate of Mrs. Oscar Johnson of the International Shoe Company of St. Louis. There was the locally famous St. Albans Inn, a prize Guernsey dairy farm, and a swimming pool, and tennis court. They needed a lifeguard, a sort of recreation director. And they would pay $40 per month, including room and board. I took the job and had it for two summers, in 1939 and 1940. It was very romantic, beautiful country, close to the Missouri River. I could have my dog, Snoopy, a wire-haired, as company. I was fed like a king. I could date who I wanted, though I had no automobile. I could invite my friends to visit me. I could hitch a ride back to St Louis, some 40 miles away. As the lifeguard, I met many attractive young people, women and men. Both genders often made a play for me. I was not interested in the men, but I went along with the women.

To illustrate how luck often plays a part in the course of one's life, let me relate what happened when I waited one evening in the parking lot of the St. Albans Inn, trying to hitch a ride back to St. Louis for a two-day vacation. I succeeded in having a young couple agree to let me accompany them to St. Louis. On the way home, they had no trouble in getting me to chatter about myself. I did not know until much later that the man, Dr. David Rioch, M.D., was a highly esteemed Professor of Neuropsychiatry at Washington University, and the woman, Janet Rioch, Ph.D., was a Clinical Psychologist. They got me to tell them about my aspirations to go to medical school and become a psychiatrist. They heard me say I was a very good student, but that I did not have the financial means to attend medical school. The man volunteered that maybe he could help me. He said he was a Professor of Neuropsychiatry at Washington University School of Medicine and that maybe he could find a position for me, some sort of Fellowship that would pay me a monthly salary that might enable me to attend medical school. After interviews with the Professor and Chairman of the Department of Psychiatry, John Whitehorn, M.D., Professor Carlyle Jacobson, Ph.D., and Professor Felix Deutsch, M.D. they offered me a Josiah Macy Foundation Psychosomatic Fellowship paying $75 per month! That was good money in those days. I would be a research assistant to Dr. Deutsch and his research assistant, Dr. David Nadel, M.D.. Hot dawg! I felt I had it made!

I asked Dr. David Rioch what further college courses I should take at Washington University undergraduate school during the academic year of 1940. I noted, I told him, that many premedical students at Washington University took biochemistry, human anatomy, neuroanatomy, physical chemistry and other science courses in preparation for medical school What should I do? He wisely advised me to take all the humanities courses that I might like, for I would have all the science courses I needed after I started to go to Washington University Medical School Besides the science courses I took that last year, such as, Experimental Embryology (taught by the great Prof. Viktor Hamburger, using frog and salamander eggs) and Experimental Genetics (using Drosophila melanogaster fruit flies), I also took Art History, Expository Writing (under Prof. Dana Jensen), American Literature (with Prof Frank Webster), and European History (with the inspiring Prof. Roland Usher). And I loved them all! I could easily go into great detail about the marvelous professors and the subject matter of these courses. But that would stray away from the binding focus of this story: the memoirs of my mother.

At Washington University Medical School, at first I was not sure I would like learning at Medical School. I liked all of the sciences I had studied, and I liked the Humanities. But Medicine? I was going to Medical School with the aim of becoming a psychiatrist. I was sure I would have to learn a lot more subjects than those relevant to Psychiatry. I did not realize I was going to be exposed to some extraordinary teachers. The first year of Medical School, I lived on Wydown Avenue in a large, luxurious home with the Nathan family, serving as the substitute father (and mother) of two young boys, Emil and Peter Nathan, and provided with a full-time cook and a housemaid and an automobile to use.

How did I happen to get into that situation? Well, I had been a camp counselor for two summers at Camp Nebagamon, and I was responsible for the youngest boys in camp, the Swampers, ages 8-9, and I had to write letters to their parents weekly on how their offspring were faring at camp. I met most of the parents at the camp when they came to visit their sons. I met Emil Nathan, Senior, at the camp during his visit there. At the end of the camp season, to my surprise he called me and asked me whether I could live with his children; I would be provided an automobile and some reasonable compensation. He was the owner of a very successful wholesale liquor business, which required his traveling frequently away from home. His wife, mother of the two boys, had died–in fact, she had committed suicide. Emil Nathan Junior, the older boy, had been one of my campers. He liked me. Could I help him out? I needed the money. I could use an automobile to drive to Medical School, which was about five miles away from the home. But I had another job; the Macy Foundation Psychosomatic Fellowship, at which I would have to work during the school year while going to Medical School Could I do all these things? I decided to try to do so. Mother encouraged me to give it a try. Father acquiesced, realizing I suppose that he could not provide adequate supplemental financial support to match this opportunity. So I became part of the Nathan family, eating rather elegantly served meals in a style to which I was not accustomed, with a cook and a maid, both trying to please. Most of the time Emil Nathan Senior was not around his residence. He had remarried after the mother of the boys had killed herself. His second wife, the stepmother of the boys, had become emotionally upset, for some reason or other, and she had decided to get psychiatric treatment somewhere in Oklahoma. And so, Mr. Nathan carried on his wholesale liquor business and visited his wife frequently in Oklahoma. So the children had a surrogate father (me). And the boys' paternal grandparents visited our household rather frequently, probably in order to see how things were going and how I was doing as a substitute parent. I liked the boys, and they liked me. The younger boy, Peter, about 6 years of age, got my quiet sympathy. He often had nightmares, and I would get up and comfort him. My bedroom was next to his, and my being close by at night-time seemed to be reassuring to him. After I lived there for a week, he sometimes came to my bedside, woke me up, and told me he was scared. And of course I hugged him and reassured him. I told the maid about his waking up at night and crying, and she told me that his mother had killed herself in the nearby bathroom by cutting her wrists, and he had seen her dead body there. That helped my heart bleed for him, and I could understand why he was plagued by nightmares. Emil, age 8-9, who had been my camper at Camp Nebagamon, had already become good friends with me.

I should relate one more short story about the Nathan boys, my first sons, because it is touching, too. One afternoon when we were playing catch in the side yard of our spacious home, and really enjoying ourselves, he suddenly asked me a question that took me by surprise. "Louis," he asked, "What is a Jew?' I replied, "Don't you know?" "No," he said. "How come you want to know? "Well, Alice, the girl that lives in that house has been one of my best friends. And she told me yesterday, that her mother told her she couldn't play with me any more because I was a Jew." What an injustice, I thought. Here I was, a Christian of Protestant and Catholic heritage, getting ready to explain to a sweet Jewish boy, who was in the process of losing a second mother and whose father was being largely absent, about the irrational prejudices of our world. I gave him a straightforward explanation along the lines that those people who decided to believe that Jesus Christ, born a Jew, was the messiah and savior of mankind became Christians, and those people who decided to believe that Christ was not the messiah who was going to save mankind were Jews or practiced a different religion. I told him that the Jews were possibly right on this matter, no one knew for sure. It was certainly not an issue which should drive people apart. When it did, that was known as "intolerance" and "prejudice" which were contrary to the American Bill of Rights and Constitution. I didn't dwell on these latter details very much because I suspected they wouldn't mean much to him at that age of his life. But I emphasized that such anti-Jewish attitudes were against the laws of the United States of America. I silently cry inside as I recall these events, and I wonder how my two boys turned out in light of these cruel aspects of human beings. I know now that Peter went to Princeton, got a doctorate there, and became a very respected Clinical Psychologist. I think Emile Junior took over his father's business, but I don't know for sure. I never did share these stories with my mother, father, or brothers, for I was so busy in those days. While living at the Nathan household, I would visit the family apartment at 6000 Waterman Avenue whenever I could. Mother was always there, and she would invariably express a serious interest to learn what I was doing in Medical School and the Nathan household. After I hit the highlights on these topics, she would tell me all about what each of my brothers was doing–seeming to treat them with equal interest and concern.

On the matter of how balanced mother's love was for her sons, I think she loved us each quite equally, was familiar with our personal strengths and weaknesses, and tried to bolster each one of us through our individual vicissitudes. And she would always share with us what papa was doing and working on.

Now I reflect I was facing a rather challenging ordeal at Medical School. I can remember studying late at night after putting the boys to sleep. My heavy anatomy book (Morris, Textbook of Human Anatomy), I often took to bed and fell asleep over it. I wondered why it had to be so big and clumsy. I remember that the section on human bones and skeleton was written by Professor Terry, our Professor of Anatomy. And, at first, as I looked at him while he lectured to us, I rather wondered how a man could become so interested in mere human bones. As the Human Anatomy course progressed, I was rather intrigued, yes maybe astounded, that a specialist in human bones, such as Dr. Terry, could tell the probable sex associated with a few bones, could make a close approximation of the height of the possessor of a leg bone, and could estimate the probable age and muscular build of the owner of a these bones.

Life actually seemed very interesting and enjoyable at this time of my life. Something new was going on every moment, and I liked this tempo of life (and I still do).. At Medical School, I could not stay late in Anatomy, as some students did, to keep up with the dissection of my half of a cadaver (In those days two students were assigned to one cadaver in Anatomy.). I just had to squeeze every assignment into the time I had available, whether or not I did a complete or perfect job. In Biochemistry I had Carl and Gerti Cori, who were to become Nobel prize winners for the discovery of the Cori cycle of glucose metabolism. In Physiology I had Professor Erlanger, another Nobel prize winner. There was Professor Edmund Cowdry in Histology, Barry Wood in Medicine, Evarts Graham (a famous lung and gall bladder surgeon and Robert Ellman (a respected general surgeon and textbook author) and Brian Blades (a very skillful plastic surgeon) in Surgery, Willard Allen in Obstetrics and Gynecology, Robert Moore in Pathology. The names and faces of these professors all come back to me, and I can recall their voices and facial expressions as they lectured. I can see and hear the other medical students as they looked in those days, and the looks and smells and noises of the Medical School and associated Hospitals and Clinics. (Those memories go back more than 55 years, and they are so clear! This memory capacity makes me wonder just how does our memory work so well? Now we know that short and long-term memory have different neurochemical bases. But now I am straying away from the main story-line.)

I was not sure I was going to like medicine, for I had aimed to go to Medical School to study Psychiatry and Neurology. I found myself liking each medical basic science I took over the first two years of Medical School. In the last two years, the clinical sciences were equally attractive to me, though the sick and sometimes dying patients pulled at my heart strings.

With the second year of Medical School, Emil Nathan Senior had decided to divorce his second wife and remain more at home with his two fine sons. I returned to my parents' home to live. Around the middle of my second year, that would have been the early part of 1942, I had an argument with my father. I don't know what I walked into with papa that day; I think he must have had money worries or a disappointment of some kind. I was largely paying my own way at Medical School, with my Macy Psychosomatic Fellowship job and a student loan. The outcome of the argument was that I could not live at home any more, my father said. What triggered the argument, I really do not know or understand. I think father was angry and disappointed over something in his life, and I became the target of his wrath. Of course, I was overwhelmed, for I did not know how I was going to manage. A medical student friend of mine told me there were jobs as attendants at the St. Louis Insane Asylum that provided room and board and a modest salary. I applied, and I got an attendant's job on the night shift from 11:00 pm to 7:00 am. I was told that after my chores of checking on patients, giving them medications, changing the sheets of incontinent patients, keeping my eyes on patients so they would not get into fights with one another, helping patients who had epileptic seizures, and so forth, that the senior attendant on the ward or floor would not object if I fell asleep at my desk or studied my books. The Asylum was large, smelly, and crowded with patients, maybe over 500 patients. On the night shift, cockroaches would come out and crawl on the walls near me or on my desk. I was allowed to put a sheet over my chair and desk so that I could spot them and brush them away. I had trouble sleeping, and my sleep was plagued by frightening nightmares. Some of the regular attendants with whom I worked were impatient, angry, and violent with patients who moaned or howled during the night. I heard and saw some of these attendants go into a ward of insane patients and if a patient did not stop howling or raving the attendant would hit him! I could not believe it! But I saw it happen frequently. After a while I did not want to see it happen. But I could hear it happen. Now I wondered did I really want to become a psychiatrist? I had never seen anything so sadistic and inhuman. A psychiatrist at this mental hospital explained to me that some of the attendants were ex-patients. But I never found out whether the ex-patients were the good attendants or the bad ones.

Somehow during this period of 4 or 5 months while I held this job and lost a lot of sleep, I was on the Obstetrics and Gynecology clinical clerkship and rotation, and instead of being very tired, I became turned on, mildly hypomanic, able to survive with only a few hours sleep per night. The experience did not seem to interfere with my capacity to learn and my grades.

And then mother got in touch with me and told me that I could come home and live there. Father had reconsidered and decided that it was all right for me to live at home. Naturally, I enthusiastically accepted this opportunity. I liked living at home. I was not unused to father having an occasional loss of temper. I respected all of his skills highly, and I had come to realize that making a livelihood as a musician, artist, composer, and newspaper journalist was difficult. Mother paved the way for my return home, and she explained to me that father had over-reacted and had, himself, felt ashamed of sending me away from home. So I came home, and I never discussed the argument and the ensuing situation again with either my father or my mother. I worked diligently at Medical School and at my Fellowship, through my freshman, sophomore, junior, and senior years. During the latter two years, the USA got into World War II. Medical students were deferred from immediate military service. During my senior year, we were put in the ASTP (I forget what it stands for), put on military duty while we attended Medical School, and we were all paid a small salary. My financial worry days were over. I now had sufficient money for modest living expenses and to pay my tuition. I graduated from Medical School December 1943 with scholastic honors and was made a member of the Medical School Scholastic Honorary organization known as Alpha Omega Alpha. I was honored to acquire an Internship in Straight Medicine at Barnes Hospital, Washington University School of Medicine, with the grand salary for the first year of $10.00 per month, room, board, and white uniforms. These years of medical internship and, later, residency, during World War II, were reduced to nine-month periods each so that we could be more rapidly trained to be available for military service during World War II, as physicians. I was such an enthusiastic and, I guess, hard-working straight-medicine intern that the

Chairman of the Department of Medicine, Professor Barry Wood, invited me to continue training as a resident physician in Internal Medicine. And the Chairman of Surgery, Professor Evarts Graham, invited me to become a resident physician in Surgery, especially Orthopedic Surgery. These famous Professors were rather surprised to be turned down in their invitations to me; I stuck to my premedical school decision to seek training as a neuropsychiatrist and become a resident physician in Neuropsychiatry under the Chairmanship of the distinguished Professor John Whitehom and, later, Professor Edwin Gildea. So the second year of post medical school education (a nine-month period), I became a resident in Neuropsychiatry, receiving $25.00 per month. And the third year as a Resident in Neuropsychiatry, I was awarded $50.00 per month. And the fourth year, I was granted, as Chief Resident in Neuropsychiatry, the grand sum of $75.00 per month. At that salary I figured I had a good enough income, along with the fine salary of my fiancee ($100.00 per month) of Dr. Helen Clarissa Reller, Chief Resident in Dermatology at Washington University School of Medicine, to get married. The marriage was held on August 24, 1944 at Centenary Methodist Church in St. Louis, Missouri.

At my Neuropsychiatric residency and Helen's Dermatology residency we were already programmed to become "workaholics." We were underpaid and overworked. And we didn't know it. In fact, we liked our work And we expected to be awakened several times during the night to handle some urgent medical calls at our hospitals. How I was able to romance this fine woman, let alone find her, during our busy times, I don't know. Maybe I was just lucky. I was very much attracted to her–for her beauty, brains, and wonderful personality. Somehow we managed to find time to become acquainted, and she returned my affection for her. I liked her parents, and she liked mine, especially my mother. I think she was somewhat awed by my father, as we perhaps all were. At my home, he performed on the piano, violin, showed his paintings, and did most of the talking at our dinner table. I didn't think that was surprising, for I was used to this. I will admit that I was rather proud of his accomplishments. Helen told me many years later what an unusual and gifted and talkative person she thought he was. She, also, ventured to say he monopolized the family conversation.

I could dwell for days and weeks here on Helen, our first encounter, our courtship, our nearly fifty years of a marvelous marriage, but I have to remind myself this essay is entitled "Memoire of My Mother." I can say that my love for Helen, my capacity to care and appreciate Helen and other women, my devotion to her and my three daughters all were shaped by my experiences with my mother. Other fine women, such as my Aunt Annie Mutrux, wife of my mother's brother, Louis, supermother of 12 children and Minerva and Marie Nott, older cousins through the Mutrux line, and others, helped me perceive the infinite good in women, helped me focus on their virtues more than their ordinary frailties.

Those war-years as "house officers" at the great Washington University Medical Center, ranging for me from January 1, 1944 through June 30, 1946, were filled with medical work and learning. I only infrequently saw and communicated with my family of origin. I only occasionally saw my parents briefly, sometimes on Holidays. Now I had another family with whom to socialize, the Reller family, Helen's parents and her younger brother, Charles. Helen's father, Harry , who had been Paymaster at Granite City Steel Company, was a 33rd degree Mason, and her mother, Frieda, was an officer in the women's counterpart of the Masons. Charlie Reller studied Civil Engineering at Washington University. He did a tour of duty in the U.S. Army during World War II. Frieda Reller was a sweet woman and mother. I can understand why she gently scolded me for getting her daughter pregnant with a second child, Claire, following the birth of my son Guy in Texas, where I was stationed as a US Public Health Service Officer, at the USPHS Hospital, in Fort Worth, Texas. Here was this sweet daughter of hers who had spent years getting educated and becoming a first-rate dermatologist. Was it right for Helen's husband, that upstart Louis, to impregnate her daughter and to enchain her to child care? From my point of view, Frieda did not realize I was devoted to Helen and to having a good-sized family. At the same time, I wanted very much to have Helen realize all of her knowledge and skills as a physician, and I wanted Helen to achieve as much professional fulfillment as a physician specialist as I. She had always been an honor student, and she was elected to Phi Beta Kappa for her good grades and to Alpha Omega Alpha (Medical School Scholastic Honorary Society). Helen's mother died in her 50's from an ovarian cancer. Harry Reller lived a long life, and he and I became very good friends. He spent much time with us when we lived in Potomac, Maryland, when I was the first Research Psychiatrist at the National Institute of Mental Health in Bethesda, Maryland. When I built a brick retaining wall for a patio in our back yard, Harry helped me; he mixed the cement while I laid the brick. I visited the first house I owned on Persimmon Tree Road in Potomac, Maryland, on that one-acre lot, in the back yard, I saw the brick wall still there (after 45 years!) that Harry and I built together. To me it signified the emotional bonding with Helen and her father. Harry Reller often visited us in Cincinnati, Ohio, where I was Research Professor of Psychiatry at the College of Medicine, University of Cincinnati, and Helen was a Professor of Dermatology. I know he had a good and positive effect as a role-model on my son Guy, who often speaks admiringly of his maternal grandfather. Too bad Frieda Reller did not live longer, for my children did not get to know her. She was devoted to her husband and two children and could have served as a role-model. Helen served that role, however, very well.

What about my mother? Mother lived to be 73 years old. She died March 8, 1953 of cancer of the colon. I was at the National Institute of Mental Health in Bethesda, Maryland from about July 1951 to July 1953, for I moved to Cincinnati, Ohio, to become Research Professor of Psychiatry in the Department of Psychiatry at the Cincinnati General Hospital and University of Cincinnati College of Medicine. She did visit us once while we were living in Chicago, Illinois (from 1948 to 1951). One of those summers (August 1950), we took a vacation to Quebec Province in Canada. I do not recall how we located the place, but it was on Lac Simon, Cheneville, Quebec. I just now found some photographs of us, showing mother, Helen, and our children. We had a little son, Guy, almost 3 years of age (born September 12, 1947), and a baby girl, Claire (born May 16, 1949). I remember driving the car through Toronto and onto Montreal. We vacationed on this lake (Lac Simon) in lower Quebec Province. It was a rural area, and English was rarely spoken and not at all by the storekeepers in the small nearby village. Mother enjoyed speaking French with them, and I enjoyed hearing the French and trying to understand what they were saying. My speaking knowledge and skill in French are fairly good, but I remember I had trouble understanding this rural Quebec French. Mother did not seem to have trouble understanding it, and she certainly helped us select and buy food. She was so good and helpful with our little children! She loved Helen and Helen loved her. We were extraordinarily congenial adults on that trip. Somehow I remember carrying two chamber pots in the back of our automobile and having to stop the car often so that the kids could use them. What an odd thing to remember. But, then, parenting has many different phases and responsibilities. And eating, sleeping, and going to the pot were big features for that developmental stage of life.

I have rather postponed mentioning it, but, unexpectedly as it often happens, I was informed by my father that mother was in the hospital (Barnes Hospital, where Helen and I had been house officers) and had cancer of the colon. I worried that it was bad, for my maternal grandmother had died of colon (rectal) cancer. I remember visiting her in the hospital. My brother Edmond said he did not want to visit her there. He said that since I was a doctor it would not bother me. He was right only in that I could cover up my fears and impending grief; I wish I could erase the visual images of my seeing her in a hospital bed. I read the hospital record and the surgical report gave her no hope. She was rather stoic. Maybe she was covering up or under the influence of a pain-killing drug. Now I wish we could have talked about what was happening to her and that we could have cried together and that I could tell her what a wonderful and inspiring mother she was. I would like to believe that she already knew how I felt about the love I had for her. I suspect she did not want to stir up our emotions. I wish we had said our farewells. But I have to reflect that she may not have known that she was going to die. I do not know whether father or her doctor told her. I did not, for I had the vain hope she might recover and survive. As I said before, she died March 8, 1953, after I had returned to Potomac, Maryland.

In a way, writing these memoirs of my mother help resolve my grief over her passing away and at the same time help me articulate, yes put into words, what a marvelous mother she was.

POSTSCRIPT

I overlooked an important detail in writing these Memoirs of My Mother. Something I did not realize until long after mother's passing away and after I had been a practicing psychiatrist for many years. In rearing her sons, mother always made herself available at different stages of our development to come up with suggestions or advice on how to cope with whatever current problem we were encountering. In the same position in my professional role with my medical and neuropsychiatric patients, I momentarily reflect on the possible solutions to the dilemmas and problems with which my patient is faced. Then, secondarily, I may ponder about where I got such a good therapeutic idea. Quite often I have come to realize that the idea originated, of course in a different context, with my mother and less so my father.

Some of these gems are: (1) A soft answer turneth away wrath. (2) If you don't succeed at first, try try try again. (3) You can do anything you put your mind to. (4) If you're upset about a problem, try considering what difference it will make in a hundred years. (5) Do unto others as you would have them do unto you. (6) Most of the time it is wise to forgive your enemies, though you may never forget.

I realize that these ideas are not original and are very old. Their survival and longevity indicate that human problems have not changed over millenia, and these remedial approaches are often of avail. And some wisdom has developed and been passed along through the generations on how to help the members of the human race get along with one another and how to deal with the vicissitudes of life on our planet. My personal experiences certainly support the position that we learn how to cope with life's problems through the words and behaviors of our parents. Thanks mother and father.

A Voyage to Europe with Claire—My Eldest Daughter

August 30, 1985

Because she had never been to Europe, as had my two other daughters, I decided to take Claire with me on a trip to Europe to visit some (mainly Mutrux) relatives. And after being invited to lecture in Hamburg and Munich, Germany. I wrote a journal during the trip and here follows my journal notes, now rather amusing and entertaining in some respects and surprisingly detailed about food, eating, Claire's shopping experiences, driving the European roads, and restaurants.

I departed with Claire from Los Angeles via Lufthansa (DER Charter) at 1:40 p.m. to Frankfurt. The plane was a DC 10, very cramped for leg space. Claire was on the window-side and I was in the middle. On my right sat an obese woman, age 69, married to an 83 year old retired electrical engineer, living in Downey, California; both she and her husband were born in Ulm, West Germany. She was returning to Ulm for her biennial visit to her four sisters. Her mother had died one year ago at age 92. She kept speaking to me in German rather than English. Very talkative. I understood three-fourths of what she said. She had one offspring, a son 34 who had studied Physics (got a B.A.) and had no job.

Both women (Claire and the woman on my right) were unable to sleep on the flight which was very smooth. I slept about two to three hours. We arrived in Frankfurt on time, and reset our watches nine hours later than California time. The flight took ten hours 45 minutes.

After getting our luggage, we found the auto-rental counter (Sixt), and we were given a four-door brown Opel Kadette rather than a two-door Fiesta, which was bigger. We drove to Metz, France uneventfully and found our hotel, a Sofitel. Quite comfortable.

Claire was delighted with our first French city. There was the Mirabell Festival for three days (mirabell = a yellow prune plum). We saw some marvelous Madagascar brown street dancers and an impressive Gothic church.

We drank beer at an outside brasserie, then bought two Monsieur le croques, cheese, cakes and soda for the road.

AUGUST 31

We left Metz and drove to Paris. We thought we had reservations for Hotel Gay-Lussac, because the woman at the Reception Desk at the Hotel Sofitel in Metz said she made the reservation "complet" (which I took to mean "complete."). It turned out that the rooms at the Hotel Gay-Lussac were, indeed, "complet" which the desk clerk at the Hotel Gay-Lussac told me were "filled" and that we had no reservations there.

Meanwhile, the acute traffic in Arr. Five was terrible. There were no parking places on the street, and many autos were parked on the sidewalk. I found a place to park on the sidewalk. I kept recalling that the auto insurance was $500 deductible. It seemed to me impossible that on Rue St. Jacquest and its surroundings that I wouldn't get hit or scraped. And, now, we had no hotel reservations! We kept driving looking for hotels on the thoroughfare we were taking, and we could see none except for the side streets, where we could sometimes see a hotel. Heading north on Rue Richard-Lenore, we spotted a hotel sign. Hotel Meridional. There we found accommodations for two nights, "une chambre avec un lit et un canape qui deplie."

We unpacked and got instructions from the female desk clerk on how to use the Metro, bought two "carnets," giving us ten rides each. We first found our way, by Metro, to LePrintemp. Claire shopped for 1.5 hours and bought two sweaters (@$147.00=1220 Francs).

I went via the escalator to the ninth floor where there was a roof garden, and I had a Pepsi and piece of cake. The view of the city was magnificent.

Then we visited the Eiffel Tower, again via Metro, and went to the very top. We tried to find a restaurant for supper, but they were closing. It was too late--11:00 p.m.. We had pieces of cheese, pretzel sticks, and soda for supper in our room.

SEPTEMBER 1, 1985

"Petit dejeuner" in room.

Then we visited a large outdoor market near the Becquet-Sabin Metro stop. Later we visited the Louvre and Notre Dame. Then we went to see Giselle Mutrux and Patrice Landau.

As I said before, we went to the neighborhood market, and then we took the Metro and saw the classic oil paintings of David depicting historical scenes (e.g., the Pope's Coronation of Napoleon I), examples of Roman sculpture (e.g., Agrippa), and Egyptian antiquities. We ate some snacks at an outdoor cafeteria on a ledge of the Louvre overlooking a courtyard that was being remodeled and in the process of reconstruction.

Then, we proceeded to Giselle's at 14 La Rue Regrattier. After ringing at 2430, the door latch of the beige metal door with a big knocker buzzed, and we entered a cobblestoned passage-way leading to a small exquisite court-yard. There were doorways to four small apartments. One was Giselle's, one was George's, one was Patrice's, one belonged to an American with property in Napa Valley who lived six months out of the year in Paris.

Giselle led us into a cramped kitchen with places for only two to sit, occupied also by a short haired moderate-sized dog and two Siamese cats, one with a stub tail. She introduced us to Patrice Laudau, a nice looking Frenchman who looked similar to Marston (a son-in-law at that time) in his face and some facial expressions.

Reluctantly, she asked whether there was anything we wanted to drink. We said we would have some tea. Over the next 15 minutes she prepared and began to pour it into blue bowls that made me wonder whether this was suppose to be some kind of soup. I discovered--with careful eye-searching--that the stylish soup bowls were actually tea cups of a striking shape.

Patrice was very talkative, and he and I chatted in French about many things. He wound up telling me about his business, frame and print-making, and saying that he had 70 "employees" in the USA.

Also, he said he wanted to show me some photos he took of cousins George and Paul. He led us to the apartment's small living room which had a very musty smell and was expensively furnished and proceeded to show us a Sony video, one that recorded and played back video on a small cassette.

The cats animals were impertinent and demanded attention, climbing all over the furniture, people's laps, and on tables.

Later, we ate at a Brasserie. Claire ate the same dish Giselle did and Patrice ordered "choucroute, jambon, and saucisse." I ate "cassouolet." Then, Patrice helped us find our way to Rue Richard-Lenoir on which we walked to our Hotel Meridional.

September 2, 1985

We left Hotel Meridional, looking for the Boulevard Peripherique to take us out of Paris towards Rouen to Trouville, France. After plugging along in some traffic jams in Paris and missing our turn-off, we found our way and got to A-13, a good toll expressway. We sailed along at 120-160 km/hr; we stopped to have a light lunch at a "Restop."

We had lots of trouble finding George's house on 49 Rue de la Cavee. The street signs were rare and hard to find and the streets were winding and narrow. We barely missed finding the street several times; a kind man driving a Honda conducted us to it.

At George's we were given rooms--livable--on the third floor.

We met Laurence, age 17, as tall as Tracy, but heavier, and with blue eyelashes. We met her boyfriend, Thierry, age 23, a boat worker, good-looking, and polite.

George looked thin but hardy; he had a lined face. He was working on rebuilding a kitchen and a covered back porch to the house. The house bore a plaque on the front door saying it had been the house of a lieutenant commander who had been the bodyguard of Napoleon I. The plaque said this homeowner had been born in the 1700's and died in the 1850's.

The house was sandwiched in between two equally old houses not bearing plaques reporting previous dwellers.

The kitchen and a dining room were on the ground floor and there was a dumb-waiter going to the first floor, which was compresed of a living room and a parlor. On the floor where Claire and I stayed, really the fourth floor, there were four small bedrooms and a bathroom. Above this floor was a small attic reached by very steep steps.

We gave Laurence and Thierry a sweatshirt with San Francisco written on the front, which Laurence loved. She was going back to Paris for a day or two. She had lost one job and had gotten another one in a Chamber of Commerce office in Deauville; she got the job because she was bilingual, i.e., French and English.

We asked George to take us to a good French restaurant. He did so. It was 23-km from Trouville. It featured the nouvelle cuisine. Claire, I, and George loved the food.

I drove home in the rain.

September 3, 1985

I spent the day chatting with George and shopping in Trouville and Deauville, adjoining coastal villages on the French side of the English channel in Normandy.

These two small towns are populated with native French people and tourists largely from other parts of France, many of whom have second residences in these townships according to George.

We had drinks in the early afternoon in a very posh resort hotel in Deauville, and then we drove out to the quay and took photos of the surf, running into Deauville, and of boats in a large boat anchorage.

We ate at a Chinese (maybeVietnamese) restaurant in Trouville--much to our liking.

September 4, 1985

After making our farewells to George, he escorted us out of the street maze of Trouville and Deauville by having us follow his car. (He said, incidentally, he planned to come to the USA in October 1985).

Then Claire and I began to drive to Freiburg, Germany. The countryside in France along the A-4 and A-36 expressways was beautiful. We were tempted to stop at several places to explore, e.g., Versailles, Fontainbleau, etc. but we refrained from so doing in order to reach Freiburg at a reasonable time. (I privately reflected that my father told me that his half-brother—a Gottschalk and a physician—had gone from the United States of America to visit Freiburg briefly before the USA got into World War I and had stayed and died in Freiburg. I wondered whether I could trace his relative.)

The only big trial of the day was to reach Uwe Koch by phone at his place of work. I tried to do so on a telephone west of Paris on the auto expressway. It was an automatic one. I couldn't figure out how to use it, and two people working at this auto stop also did not know how to phone Germany.

At another restop, with the help of a French telephone assistant, I finally reached Uwe Koch. He gave me his home address: 6A Schlierburg Strasse. He told me to phone him after we reached the Center of Freiburg, and he would come to meet us and escort us to his house.

All that happened as planned. And then we had a fine meal prepared by Trixie Koch.

SEPTEMBER 5, 1985

I discovered I was scheduled to give a lecture and workshop in the Department of Rehabilitation Psychology at Albert Ludwig University around 9:30 a.m. I got up early and found some slides to fortify my presentation.

There were about a dozen people attending the presentation. Uwe gave a brief 10 minute introduction of me and my subject matter, in German, as planned. I spoke in English for about one hour and, then, responded to questions, for about 30-45 minutes.

After this session some of us went to a special room for videotaping group therapy where we were served coffee. Some of the people remained and another discussion was initiated by Uwe regarding the activities of my Psychiatry Consultation and Liaison Division as well as the nature and range of my private psychiatric practice and the kind of psychotherapy I use. I said what I always say under such questioning---that I tailor my psychiatric treatment to the patient and the problem rather than trying to tailor the patient to my technique of psychiatric treatment.

After a lunch with Uwe in which I had a beer and Fleischkase and white or dark bread (without butter), Uwe took me to his office and painstakingly he went through every chapter of the book on the Gottschalk-Gleser scales of which he is the senior editor (Gert Schofer is junior editor). He estimated there were over 800 pages in this book, which will be published in German by Beltz Verlag out of Weinheim, Germany.

I was overawed by the scope and quality of over 30 original papers using the Gottschalk-Gleser scales, primarily those involving the measurement of anxiety and hostility. Uwe gave me a frontispiece and table of contents. I wrote a Foreword for the book and a chapter reviewing non-German studies. The book is scheduled to come out in the fall or winter of 1985.

At 4:00 p.m. Uwe had to be at a Kurklinik. He drove me there in our rental car--an Opel Kadette--so that I could find my way back to his home at 6A Schlieberg Strasse while he attended patients at the Kurklinik. He introduced me to a Dr. Kamper, the Medical Director of the Klinik, who showed me around the place. Uwe walked around with us to explain some of the details because my host, Dr. Kamper, had some deficiencies in his knowledge of English.

The Kurklinik has a capacity to house 100 patients. The average length of stay is four weeks. The patients are not psychotic but do have medical or post-surgical problems or mental problems. The care program is something like a half-way house or an ambulatory care nursing home. The therepy provided include physiotherapy, massage water treatment in the form of various kinds of baths, massage exercise, swimming, fishing, occupational therapy, meditation, and psychotherapy.

The physical facilities were beautiful, the surroundings were tastefully landscaped and included plenty of flowers. The equipment and the therapy rooms and patients' rooms--all private--were absolutely spotless and technically new and modern. I kept thinking of the term "scrubby dutch."

I was told the use of medicaments is minimized--but utilized--here. I have never seen anything comparable in the USA. The doors, drawers, and other fittings were reminiscent of the elegant level of the mechanics of a Mercedes-Benz. Walls and cabinet doors were white or very light gray or brown. Colorful modern pictures decorated the walls.

I asked Uwe how much the Medical Director might be paid. He estimated $3,000 marks/month. He casually asked the Medical Director what his salary was in German, remarking I had asked and what he had estimated and the Medical Director matter-of-factly replied he received less. But on further questioning by me, he acknowledged he was allowed to do private-practice.

I drove back to Uwe's house and took a much needed 1-2 hour nap and then, returned to the Kurklinik to pick up Uwe and bring him home. It was raining lightly.

We ate a delicious cold supper at the Koch's home composed of cheeses, smoked trout, small shrimp, German breads, champagne and white wine.

Uwe and I chatted until midnight. Claire and Trixie chatted with us too, but retired earlier--about 11:00 p.m.

SEPTEMBER 6, 1985

Claire and I slept later than the Kochs. We could hear their two children gamboling around in their apartment. They are fraternal twins, and 2 ½ years of age. They are both blond. The boy (Milan) has dark brown eyes and the girl (Lil) has light blue eyes.

We went out shopping with Corinne (a 27-year-old half-sister of Trixie) and I was shown around the middle of the City of Freiburg by Dr. Michael Bodar and Dr. Uwe Koch. I learned it had been severely bombed during the latter part of World War II--the early I940's--and has been completely rebuilt to preserve the original style of the 200-400 year old building. It was beautifully picturesque and spotlessly clean.

We met Claire and Corinne in the Munster Market and had a lunch of quiche and a glass of local white wine that had a heady flowery-like bouquet and a gentle light taste. I could quickly detect in 5-10 minutes its subtly intoxicating effects.

We returned to Uwe's home; Trixie had to return to work. Shortly, as planned, Uwe drove us in the Opel Kadette to Breisach, Germany, near the French border, then to Colmar, France, to something on a hill that looked like a medieval castle that turned out to be a "munster"--another fine gothic church, featuring an exquisite 16th century huge wood carving of the crucifixion and some stained glass windows having a geometrical abstract design depicting no human figures.

In Columar, we tramped about the beautiful medieval town, amazed at all the people walking about shopping. Most were stylishly dressed. Claire said the women's clothing in the stores and on the backs of people were very smart and fashionable.

We treated ourselves to a framboise glace and later to one chocolate truffle each.

And then Uwe drove us to an ancient walled town--surrounded by vineyards, as all these towns and cities seem to be--with cobblestones. Again we were surprised that this town, Riquewihr, not on our road map, was full of tourists, mostly from France or Germany. Claire was wearing her newly purchased soft leather boots, and they went click-click-click on the cobblestones, and she said her toes were beginning to hurt. She even confided she was becoming sight-seeing weary.

Nevertheless we hobbled around up a cobblestone street. And we went through an ancient torture chamber at three French francs apiece.

On driving back to Freiburg, Uwe got lost on the narrow rural roads. He found his way back to Colmar, France, and the rest of the drive home was easy. In the comfortably warm weather and the perfumed wine fields, Claire and I briefly dozed off while Uwe drove home.

I took us all out to a splendid supper at the Traube Restaurant in Freiburg. The food and white wines were memorable. It was a five-course fish meal for three of us. Claire had beef steak. It was not quite as good as the one we had with George Mutrux at the Dolphin Restaurant 28 kilometers from Deauville, France, but good. The "rechnung" totalled 329 German marks (the exchange rate that day was one American dollar =2.83 German marks). This was the very highest restaurant charge thus far. Good thing I had a credit card to use, so I didn't have to worry about expenses.

SEPTEMBER 7, 1985

This was Saturday, and we all got up later than usual. Typically, I got up earlier than the others and showered and bathed and wrote in this journal.

Breakfast was, as usual, with the two little children, Milan, a brown-eyed fraternal twin boy, and Lil, a blue-eyed fraternal twin girl. They sat in high chairs and chatted contently while their mother and father talked and served them, or others. We had fruit juice, coffee, German or French breads and rolls, butter, pates, cheeses, and marmalades or honey.

This day it was planned that Claire and Trixie would go shopping in Freiburg. Uwe and I were to go with Milan and Lil to the country, though we could have gone to Freiburg with the woman to shop also. Both Uwe and I preferred to go to the country. He drove my Opel, with the children in the back sucking pacifiers, to Kaiserstuhl, some low mountains that are suppose to look like a chair for the Kaiser. We drove through manicured vineyards, back and forth up a medium-sized hill, and we came to a pleasant Inn overlooking an attractive valley of grape orchards. Behind a fenced enclosure there were chickens, geese, and ducks, and a goat, which the children watched and admired. The kids were bought popsicles by Uwe. We got green sweet grapes covered with ice cream, whipped cream, and topped with two cookies. The children seemed to know Uwe would give them his cookies on request. They did not ask for mine.

Uwe told me about a graduate student of his who developed meningo-encephalitis after an insect bite, and he is now crippled, but of sound mind. Uwe is having him score five minute speech samples already collected—so he does not have to ambulate much--on the social alienation-personal disorganization scale. This student will do his dissertation on this scale, translating it into German and carrying out some kind of investigation with it. I gave him some suggestions and referred him to a couple of our papers about using this scale about which he might not know. German papers involving the Gottschalk-Gleser scales that have come out under his jurisdiction have all been of high scientific calibre. So I expect some excellent new German studies to be produced using the social alienation-personal disorganization scale and, possibly, the cognitive impairment scale.

This afternoon we lazed around the house. I saw Claire's pretty clothing purchases, a silk skirt, blouse, and vest, which she told me were almost half the price the some creations would cost in the USA.

Uwe invited me to watch television with him to see some sport shows. We saw several sports-events, including Munich playing Hamburg in soccer.

Tonight, we were invited to accompany our hosts to a large wedding reception beginning at 8:00 p.m. and lasting very late. Claire and I were delighted to go though we planned to leave early the next day on the first leg of our trip to Hamburg. Uwe has kindly arranged for us to stay in the apartment of some friends, Dr. Cristoph Schmeling-Kludas and Dr. Christiane Kludas, who live in Eppendorf near the University of Hamburg. He called and cancelled the reservations made by Dr. Adolph Meyer at the Hotel Basler Hospiz.

The wedding reception was informal. The reception was very crowded with people, mostly academic and professional types. The bride was a psychiatrist doing graduate work in "rehabilitation psychology." The groom was a professor of something.

Buffet served food included salads, ham, fleischkase, potato salad (yum), red currants with whipped cream topping. Beer and wine flowed generously.

There was dancing from audio-cassettes.

I spoke to a neuropsychologist who was a neurologist (Wellisch), a medical historian who was a pediatrician (Seider), another medical historian who had written extensively on the history of psychotherapy before Freud (Schott), a speech therapist, a gymnasium teacher, and so forth.

I even danced with Trixie, an enthusiastic dancer.

Claire was beautiful in her new skirt, blouse, and vest. But she got abdominal cramps, and we came home at a time that was considered early, 11:30 p.m.

SEPTEMBER 8, 1985

Claire told me she was ill all night with chills and fever, diarrhea, and abdominal cramps. She said she felt well enough to drive to Gottingen. I didn't have any antibiotics, nor did she. She loaded up with Lomotil and aspirin.

After farewells to the Koch family, including two kisses from each of the Koch children, we started off to Gottingen, with Uwe driving our auto to pick up his car which had been left at the place of last night's wedding because Trixie had too much to drink to drive home, according to Uwe. On the way, we stopped to get some gasoline because the tank of our car was almost empty. At the filling station we discovered we were missing the key to open the gas tank cap. What could we do now? I suddenly remembered that I had seen a loose key on Uwe's desk where I customarily placed the car keys at his home. Maybe that was our missing gas-tank cover key? Uwe drove back to his home, and I located the key. We made our farewells all over again to the Kochs. Uwe, then, drove us to his car, and from it he escorted us through the winding complex maze of Freiburg's streets to the autobahn.

I drove uneventfully to Gottingen while Claire drowsed and slept off and on for 5-6 hours. The Lomotil and the gastrointestinal disorder put her out of the picture. By the time we got to Gottingen she was beginning to feel better and more alert.

She selected Gebharts Hotel from the Michelin guide and after a few mistakes in finding our way to it on Goethealleestrasse--a problem we were getting accustomed to encountering in German cities and towns for a number of reasons, we found our choice of a hotel in Gottingen. What luck—there was a room at what was supposed to be the best hotel in town.

It did, indeed, turn out to be very comfortable. It had a "schwimmenbad," indoors and heated. Our bedroom was large with an adjoining sitting area, television, and an elegant bathroom.

Claire lay down to drowse and sleep some more, and I went out to walk and explore exercise after the long 350 mile drive. Gottingen is an old famous University town, full of shops, restaurants, and people on the street. I took a long invigorating walk and located a Ratskeller that accepted, American Express credit cards and marked it in my mind as our place to eat supper.

When I came back to the hotel Claire was still asleep. So I took a swim in the pool. That was delightful!

We went to the chosen Ratskeller Restaurant. Poor Claire was feeling better and had tomato soup and some breaded meat on toast. I had a delicious whole fish with potatoes and salad plus German beer. I gobbled down every bit of my meal and finished what Claire did not eat.

We came home and phoned Helen and Ray (Claire's husband).

SEPTEMBER 9, 1985

In the morning we had breakfast (fruhstuck) in the hotel's dining room.

When signing out from the Gebhards Hotel, I was comforted to see the hotel charge, including breakfast was 165 marks. But the charge for the phone calls to Helen and Ray was around 231 marks! Over $80.

Claire was definitely mending from her gastrointestinal ailment--we guessed it must have been something she ate. We took turns driving to Hamburg. Following Uwe's carefully drawn diagrams and the Michelin maps of Hamburg, we pointed our way to Kaffee Haus Eldor on Eppendorferstrasse or 137 Erikistrase. The former location was where we were to meet, at 1:00 p.m., Ingrid Rieman and/or Gerhart Deffner, who would guide us to 137 Erikastrasse where we would find the apartment of Dr. Cristoph Schmeling-Kludas and Dr. Cristiane Kludas. Uwe Koch had arranged for us to stay at this apartment of his Hamburg friends who were in Italy for 2-3 months. Uwe cancelled the hotel reservations for us in Hamburg that had been made by Dr. Adolph Meyer.

How got through the maze of Hamburg streets--not quite being able to follow Uwe's diagram--and actually locate the Kaffee Haus Eldor, an inconspicuous place, and meet both Ingrid and Gerhard at 1:00 p.m. I do not know. We did.

We had coffee with them. They led us to 137 Erikastrasse, which was a nice large apartment. Obviously the couple had a little child.

Clair started the washer and dryer. It blew a fuse!

The water was cold. An upstairs neighbor showed us how to turn on the water heater. And although I guessed we may have blown a fuse, and found the fuse and replaced it, the neighbor confirmed that was the problem and got the dryer and washer working again.

The apartment was cold, and we couldn't find the right key to open a basement door where the gas furnace was supposed to be located.

I invited Gerhart and Ingrid to have dinner with us. Incidentally, they were very good looking people, light-complexioned of course, in their early thirties. Uwe said Ingrid lived in one of the rooms of Gerhart's apartment and probably had been lovers at one time, but they were not so anymore. Ingrid declined my offer. Gerhart thought for a moment and accepted, saying he would bring his girlfriend.

Gerhart had to return to work. Ingrid showed us around the nearby shopping district and then departed after pointing out an Italian restaurant where we might have lunch.

Claire was, certainly, feeling better and eyed what was in the windows of antique stores.

We did have lunch at the Italian restaurant. Claire had lasagna, and I had spaghetti with fish, little shrimps and so forth. Boy, were both the dishes good!

We came back to our apartment and tried some more to figure out how to turn on the heat. No luck. We could not locate the right key.

At about 6:30 p.m. Gerhart came back and took us for a tour of the city, including a beautiful park on a lake where people were sailing and a grand city hall, old fashioned and baroque and completely restored. Then we went to pick up Gerhart's girlfriend, Azzisa. She was studying to be a speech therapist. Her grandfather had been an East Indian. She was perfectly beautiful--a black-haired medium- complexioned beauty. She claimed not to know much English. But later we found she spoke fairly well. Gerhart spoke such good English that she was embarrassed to speak it, Gerhart told us.

We had dinner near the Hamburg docks at a restaurant specializing in sea food. We all selected the same entree: flounder with mushrooms, onion. shrimps, and crabmeat, potatoes, and a salad. And for me and Azzisa, beer. Gerhart drank mineral water and so did Claire. I asked Gerhart why he didn't drink beer or wine? Yes, he did, he said. But he was driving and was responsible for us; so he would only drink water and nothing alcoholic.

We learned that Gerhart had hoped to be appointed an Assistant Professor in the Department of Psychology at the University of Hamburg. But though- his appointment had been approved, 80 new faculty appointments were not going to be funded. Or rather, only eight of these new appointments would be funded. He was in doubt if his would be. He had been invited to apply for a Fellowship at the University of California at Berkeley, and he had done so. But Azzisa had been one of 16 applicants out of 600 who had applied for special training in speech therapy at the University of Hamburg and, now, he was really reluctant to leave Hamburg should he get a Fellowship at the University of California, Berkeley. He confessed briefly he had never had a problem of this sort before, always previously finding it easy to come and go from a place regardless of whom he was dating. He looked sad and unsettled as he mentioned this.

Claire and I returned to our cold apartment on 137 Erikastrasse, got under warm covers and fell asleep.

SEPTEMBER 10, 1985

Claire and I woke up out of warm beds into a cold apartment. After a breakfast at home of sweet rolls we bought from a bakery in Gottingen, we decided to explore the nearby shops. Claire had considered getting her hair done and, maybe, buy some eye glasses. I agreed to go along for the walk and, ambivalently, consider purchasing a sweat or jogging suit, in part to keep me warmer.

It was an overcast day, cool, windy, and moist, similar to all the past few days we had experienced in Hamburg. We brought along raincoats and an umbrella.

Window shopping was interesting and the large variety of shops included stores for jewelry, clothes, antiques, food, hair, dresses, furniture, electronic goods and restaurants of all kinds. Among the latter were the USA's revenge on Hamburg for inventing the hamburger: *McDonalds*. We saw about three of these on our walk. I did buy a jogging suit and so did Claire. The women's clothes were diverse and elegant and some were very expensive. Claire said they came from all over Europe and not many from Germany—a phenomena resulting from the Common Market.

Claire priced some eyeglasses and found them stylish but as costly as in the U.S.A.

Claire searched for an English-speaking hair dresser and finally found one, and scheduled a hair job estimated to take 3 to 3.5 hours at a bargain-price of 75 marks because she selected an apprentice to do the job. I thought it was very expensive to be a woman, considering, also, the prices of clothes we saw in the stores.

We stopped at a restaurant to have a short lunch. We had beers, of course, a bowl of shrimp soup with a small slice of German bread--outstanding. Claire had sliced cold roast beef, some marvelous cream in a smart, little gravy pourer and some fried German potatoes. Claire wouldn't share all her fine potatoes with me. She licked her plater clean.

Claire got her hair done--a trim, coloring, and a permanent. It looked wonderful to me. But her hair had looked just about as good to me beforehand. She explained her new one would make her look different and feel different inside. She had resigned from her position as a relief charge nurse just before we started on these travels, and she was beginning a new job working for a pair of doctors in Laguna Beach. She felt she wanted to start, on her return to the USA, as a new person.

We did a bit more shopping, returned to our apartment, rested and had telephone calls from Uwe Koch and Gerhart Deffner. We learned there was nothing we could do about our cold apartment.

About 8:45 p.m. we began to have our dinner at a Sicilian restaurant off Ependorflandstrasse. We could hear German, Italian, and, at one table, Spanish spoken around us. But no French.

Claire selected scampi, and I ordered calamari. With our Hamburger-Pilz beer and our tasty meals we looked at our maps and planned a short trip to Denmark for the next day.

September 11, 1985

We headed towards Kiel and Flensburg, Germany, in our trusty Opel. I carefully chartered our way from Eppendorferlandstrasse, 137 Erikastrasse to be correct, towards Kiel, using my city map of Hamburg, my Automobile Club of Southern California map of Germany, and the Michelin guide map of Hamburg. I even drew a sketch of our exit route. This preparation was to no avail because of one-way streets, name changes of streets as they continue and so on. But big blue signs on one street indicated the KIEL autobahn was in a certain direction. We followed the signs, found the autobahn, and headed towards KIEL and FLENSBURG.

Speeding past the turn-off to Schleswig, we moved on towards Flensburg. At Fleneo sg, we did not feel hungry and so we decided to drive on to Denmark.

We went through the customs and, for the first time, while in Europe, our passports got stamped. I told the Danish passport agent, in my poor German, that we were only going to stay 2 to 3 hours and that we were tourists. He looked at our passports, smiled and said "Oh, you are Americans; go ahead."

Encouraged by his American-sounding English, I asked him whether there were places for shopping in any nearby town. Our map showed only Sonderborg and not much else of Denmark, for it was a map of Germany. He directed me to Sonderborg.

Sonderborg was about 53 kilometers from this border stop between Germany and Denmark. We found our way there easily, took photos, and ate what an English-speaking waitress said was a typical Danish lunch: trout, potatoes, and salad for me and a ground meat patty with gravy and salad for Claire. The food was not something special-- just plain food for two hungry people.

Before lunch we stopped at a gift and candy shop, and I asked the young woman—who did not not speak much English--in my halting German whether she could suggest some presents that were typically Danish for two German friends. She suggested chocolate candies. Claire and I selected two kinds, and the young woman gift-wrapped them.

In driving back from Sonderborg, we went in the wrong direction on good roads that we did not have on our poor map and ended up at FYNSHAV, from which one can continue only by ferry-boat towards Copenhagen. We drove back through rural and pastoral countryside. The houses and barns and fields and churches,too, looked different to us from those in Germany and France. Hay harvesting and baling, grazing dairy cows, thatched roofs, and a highway machine with a rotary brush cleaning a two-lane highway were some of the novelties we saw.

We found our way back to 137 Erikastrasse surprisingly easily amidst the scurrying traffic in Hamburg around 5:00 p.m. just following signs on the winding streets pointing to Eppendorf. Frequent directional signs at crossroads in the big city of Hamburg makes finding one's way by auto feasible, though I often had the odd feeling we got where we aimed to go by luck rather than by reason.

At 7:45 p.m. promptly as promised, Gerhart Deffner and Ingrid Rieman came by to take us to Adolph Meyer's home for dinner. Shortly before they arrived, I discovered two things that looked like they might solve the problem of our cold apartment: (1) a thermostat behind a door, and (2) a big door key that opened the basement door to the gas furnace for our apartment. I pushed a button on the gas furnace and a light went on and I set the thermostat. Nothing happened except little clicks here and there. Gerhart read the instructions on operating the furnace, turned on a gas valve, but said he was reluctant to go further to get the heater started because the instructions said the water level had to be up to a certain point and it was not. I asked the upstairs neighbor, Herr Rieck, whether he could start the furnace now that we had the key and he said he would try to do so after he and his wife had finished their supper.

We drove off to the Meyers' residence and they had three other guests to be introduced: Dr. Stephan Ahrens, Dr. Lamprathar, Dr Denike, all members of his Psychosomatic Department and apparently psychoanalysts. Dr. Meyer's wife and two sons were at the door to greet us. The two handsome blond boys, 17 and 11, smiled as they shook hands with me and brought their heels together in a fine gentlemanly German style. The younger boy, whom

I had met at my own home on the evening of August 27, 1985, spoke no english; so we spoke in French together. He was chewing gum. I liked both these boys. They went swimming in our pool in California. Their mother said they had to go to bed soon. At 8:30 p.m., I wondered?

Ingrid and Gerhart brought a beautiful bouquet of flowers for our host, and I offered my Danish gift-wrapped chocolate candy.

The conversation was very animated. I concentrated on talking with Adolph Meyer, and he made no effort to bring the other men into our conversation throughout and after the meal. Claire chattered with our hostess, Almuth, a charming, effervescent, attractive woman, with Ingrid, and with some of the men from time to time.

Adolph was very goal-oriented in his conversation. And this is one of the main reasons I think, we monopolized each other's company at this informal buffet dinner. He was, also, refreshingly blunt and direct about many subjects. He had just come from attending the International Congress of Psychosomatic Medicine in Chicago. He asked what I thought of:

1. Franz Alexander's contributions to psychoanalysis. He was told by Charles Kligerman of Chicago that Alexander was unorthodox in manipulating psychoanalytic patients.
2. The purported decline of psychoanalysis in psychiatry in the U.S.A.
3. The lack of scientific interest among psychoanalysts in the U. S.A. and Germany.

He threw light on matters I had not known.

1. Under his aegis, his psychoanalytic institute applied for a research grant from the German Federal government and got a 13-year grant of well over a million dollars to use the Gottschalk-Gleser scales in basic and clinical research. Dr. Hippius, Chairman of Psychiatry at the University of Munich and a biologically oriented psychiatrist, was one of the peer group members who approved the research grant.
2. He is writing, in English, a monograph on psychoanalytic interpretation involving how the psychoanalyst lines up his awareness of his counter-transference with his interpretive decisions with his analysand.
3. He does not believe Heinz Kohut wrote well or was accurate on the subject of narcissism. He believes that Otto Kernberg not only is a more clear writer than Kohut, but has a more valid concept of narcissism.
4. He does not believe most physicians have good scientific training. Hence, as psychoanalysts they do not add much to the science of psychoanalysis.
5. He thought psychologists had better training as scientists but when they get into psychoanalytic training most of them forget their science.
6. He thought the meeting of the International Congress of Psychosomatic Medicine in Chicago was mediocre: (a) Because the American president of the Congress, Chase Kimball, does not have much scientific and academic stature and (b) Chicago is not regarded as an attractive place to go for conventions.
7. I told him Chase Kimball was not a psychoanalyst. He said Kimball spent 10 years on Kohut's couch.

8. Michael Balint, with Enid Balint, came regularly to Hamburg as well as Cincinnati. He liked Balint very much. Also, Enid Balint was giving a talk in English, the evening of the very day (Friday, 9/18/85) I was talking.
9. He knew that Paul Ornstein had assumed leadership of self-psychology. Often, he observed, disciples clarify the thinking and writings of charismatic characters. He did not think Paul Ornstein, with Anna Ornstein, had done so with respect to "self-psychology." The "self" and the "psychology of narcissism" have not been clarified by the Ornsteins.
10. He is a staunch believer that only by careful content analysis and taping of sessions can a valid science of psychoanalysis and psychology be achieved.

When we returned home to Erika Strass, our apartment was warm. The neighbor upstairs, Herr Rieck, had got the heater started.

September 12, 1985

We slept very late. I got up at 8:00 a.m., Claire at 9:00 a.m. Though the day started overcast and cloudy, the sun came out later. Because nothing was scheduled for us by others, we had planned to visit the Hamburg Art Museum.

Around10:30 a.m. we pointed our Opel towards the "Centrum" and found ourselves in a crowded downtown area just where we aimed to be. We located the Haupbahnhof (Central Station) and across the street from it was the "Kunsthalle." There was an amazing exhibit of holograms. In addition, we saw an exhibit of modern masters (1700-1900) and old masters (1200-1600).

Then we ate what Claire thought was our best Hamburg lunch sitting outdoors across from the Hauptbahnhof. Starting with Pilz-Morovia beer, Claire had a stew mixture of three meats (veal, beef, and turkey) plus potatoes and salad, and I had their weekly special (eisbein and sauerkraut mit kartoffein) (pig's knuckles, sauerkraut, and potatoes).

We took a walk around the neighborhood. We lost a few marks in a "Spielkasse," one of several places with various slot machines. We passed by several places selling erotica or sexually explicit movies. And we found ourselves walking through an area of sporty-looking women that gave men very direct eye contact. Men were walking into or out of upstairs establishments. These places were nearby the respectable hotels and restaurants across the street from the Hauptbahnhof which was surrounded by many fancy tour buses.

We loafed at our apartment for the rest of the afternoon and early evening, anticipating a dinner at the home of Dr. Stephan Ahrens in the company of Dr. Gerhart Deffner. Gerhart came for us at 8:30 p.m. bringing Azzisa. The Ahrens live on Haynstrasse in a newly remodeled fine apartment of 1906 vintage. Bettina Ahrens is a tall slim good-looking woman who said she was a buyer for women's clothes for a man in Kiel, where the Ahrens own a residence. Stephan was a professor at the University of Kiel. Now he has a tenured (life–time) professorship at the University of Hamburg, Psychosomatic Division. He is a psychiatrist, psychoanalyst, and social scientist.

We were first served a drink with apricot liquor that was heavily laced with alcohol and loosened everybody up. Dinner had four courses: (1) A dish of spinach and an omelet covered with a thin slice of salmon--very good; (2) a beautifully decorated salad (made by Stephan); (3) the main course--tenderloin of beef, spinach macaroni, leeks with an elegant gravy; (4) an ice cream dish decorated with a piece of *the* Danish chocolate we brought as a present. All this was washed down with lots of marvelous French wine.

We talked and joked until about 1:30 a.m. and walked home to sober up.

SEPTEMBER 13, 1985

I awoke at 9:00 a.m. and Claire around 9:30 a.m. This was the day I was scheduled to perform at a noon-time seminar reviewing the book *The Content Analysis of Verbal Behavior in Clinical Medicine and Psychiatry* of which I was the senior editor and which is being published by Springer-Verlag out of Heidelberg, Germany. I had prepared myself to perform and to bring along, also, a set of our reprints on the application of my content analysis method to children for Dr. Margrite Kerekejarto who asked for such on visiting our home with Dr. Meyer and his family the night of August 27, 1985.

Stephan drove me to the office of Dr. Meyer at 11:30 a.m. in a VW 1979 convertible along with Bettina, Azzisa, and Claire. The women were dropped off to go shopping and have lunch.

Dr. Meyer (Dolph) showed me his new offices, conference rooms, and psychophysiology laboratory which looked impressive and quite adequate.

I was introduced to an audience of about 15-20 people in glowing terms by Adolph. I gave my talk in 50 minutes and answered some good questions. Obviously I made a good impression.

I had lunch with Dolph, Stephan, and Gerhart in a pleasant out-of-doors French restaurant. I had beer and a cream soup with bits of mint leaves and small crabmeat doughballs. Gerhart had mineral water and a salad, a dish of mushrooms. Dolph had white wine and a type of chicken salad. Stephan had white wine and some kind of fish. The wine drinkers made comments of satisfaction, in German, about the wine.

Conversation was relaxed and cheerful. Dolph has to retire from the University at 65. He will continue to practice psychoanalysis. The charges for a training analysis are 90 to 120 marks per session, and for a non-training psychotherapeutic session are 100 to 200 marks per session. Most sessions are 50 minutes. Dolph's are 45 minutes. Dolph heard that the Psychiatry Department at UCLA hires well-known retired professors. I told him more about this practice. He would not mind retiring in the USA. He gets an income from Switzerland and Germany.

Stephan took us to his apartment to meet Bettina and Claire and have a glass of afternoon champagne. We made our farewells to Bettina, and then Stephan drove us to the Aussen-Alster lake from which Claire and I walked home (>one half hour).

The cleaning lady was in the apartment, and I gave her a note in German which Uwe had written explaining our presence there. She spoke no English. She left us alone in a short time.

After a pleasant and informative phone call from Helen, Claire and I had our last supper in Hamburg at our favorite Sicilian restaurant.

SEPTEMBER 14, 1985

We got up late and prepared to leave Hamburg. There were lots of chores to do. Turn off the gas furnace in the basement, turn off the gas hot water heater in the bathroom, fold the sheets and pillowcases Uwe had lent us, dump the garbage, wash the dishes, leave a letter for the doctors Kludas thanking them for letting us be uninvited guests in their apartment, leave a 50 mark note to cover our phone calls, pack our suitcases, load the car, drop the key to the Kludas apartment at 28 Haynstrasse for Gerhart to give to Uwe Koch who was going to use the apartment in about a week. Then we had to find our way out of Hamburg and to the autobahn going towards Hanover. We made a few mistakes, but every mistake was promptly corrected.

The expressway was crowded, and we saw--going in the opposite direction--a long military convey composed of U.S. tanks, armored cars, supply trucks, medical corps trucks, and so forth. (I silently wondered what the Germans thought of the U.S. military presence in their country.) We ate lunch in Gottingen at our favorite Rathskeller in the "Zentrum" of town. Claire liked the old-world atmosphere and the food. So did I. She was surprised that what she ordered was a good-tasting stew composed of small slices of calves' livers. She didn't eat all of it because it reminded her of a cat liver she saw in a dissection. I had veal steak and little potato pancakes. The former was tasty but chewy and the latter were delicious with tiny pieces of some green vegetable in them. My meal was good, but more than I could eat.

The downtown square of Gottingen and the nearby streets were filled with people shopping and just walking or sitting. We walked by our Gebhards Hotel which we liked, and each of us said silent farewells to Gottingen, a quaint and picturesque university town.

We decided to go as far as Rothenburg ob den Tauber and bed down there. Stephan Ahrens had recommended our staying there. It was a precious walled city, 30 km off the autobahn, but crowded with tourists. We couldn't get a room at our first choice of a hotel, the Eishut. Our second choice, Hotel Goldener Hirsch, netted us a beautiful room overlooking a valley; the room was without bath or toilet, but with a washbasin. After a walking tour around the town, which was really surrounded by a great wall and a moat, we noted that the place was what Claire called "a tourist trap," full of well-stocked and expensive shops.

We dined in an absolutely delightful restaurant in our hotel, Die Blaue Terrasse where we had a real gourmet meal plus two Rothenburg brewed beers a piece.

SEPTEMBER 15, 1985

Well, this is the day we were scheduled to arrive in Munich and stay at the Hotel on der Oper at 10 Falkenturnstrasse. I could see from the map of Munich it was in the middle of the city. Actually, getting there would be a problem that I was prepared, morally, to face.

After a trip avoiding the autobahn to Nurnberg and traveling over back roads, we reached the autobahn directly to Munich via Augsburg. Claire was driving, and I did the navigating from two maps. We drove and drove after reaching the city to get to the central section. We missed a small turn off from Maximilianstrasse to our destination, a narrow street having only one-way traffic. I only asked about 3 people for directions. Only one out of the three could help. But we found the hotel. Our room was on the fourth floor, #44. There was no porter, but, thank goodness, there was an elevator. The desk clerk was--as most others in these smaller European hotels--obliged to do everything. He directed us to a restaurant specializing in French and Italian cuisine, the Austernkeller. It was superb.

It was also raining, and we could not linger at the shop windows, though we could see the products displayed were elegant and many items were expensive.

Our helpful desk clerk was tested by us to see how Claire could best reach and take a 9:15 a.m. Lufthansa Charter plane out of Frankfurt on September 19, 1985. He phoned us in five minutes and said there was a 7:15 a.m. plane out of Munich that would get her to Frankfurt one hour before departure time. That, I was afraid, was cutting it too close, and I resolved to work on this problem the next day.

SEPTEMBER 16, 1985

As I woke up I found myself working on the problem of Claire's reaching her Lufthansa Charter flight in Frankfurt to Los Angeles. I would ask Michael von Rad to have his secretary check it out, or get the help of Claudia Walther, Sue's friend in Munich. Claire agreed those were good ideas. So, I enlisted Michael's help. He had just returned to his two jobs in Munich from Chicago and, then, Italy and was resuming work in Munich this morning. All Bavaria, he said, was returning from vacation. In good spirits, he said he would ask his secretary, who was also just coming back from vacation to help us on this matter.

Our desk clerk turned out to be right. There was a 7:15 a.m. Lufthansa plane out of Munich that arrived in Frankfurt at 8:15 a.m, and Michael reassured us that would be sufficient time to make the necessary connection with the Lufthansa (DER) flight to Los Angeles. On Michael's advice, Claire called Lufthansa herself, spoke in English, and booked her flight out of Munich to Frankfurt for 7:15 a.m. on 9/19/85. Her baggage, she was told, could be shipped through to Los Angeles. I thought I had better accompany her to the Munich Airport to see that everything got off okay and, of course, to pay for her flight.

Michael invited us to have dinner with him and his family in Feldkirch this evening, and he recommended we take the 5-6 train to get there, leaving Marienoplatz station at 7:21 p.m. and arriving at 8:38 p.m.--typical German concepts of punctuality.

I also reached Claudia, and she asked us to join her for dinner the next evening.

Claire and I walked around our neighborhood in the middle of Munich after breakfast with a couple in their late fifties from New Jersey who had traveled fairly much in Europe. He had a son who graduated from the University of Virginia Medical School at Charlottesville and was doing a residency in North Carolina in Family Practice. They were driving to Italy and Yugoslavia tomorrow.

Claire found our neighborhood surrounded by fascinating clothing shops and gift shops. I found it interesting too. A historic City Hall (Rathaus), many people, a national theater, a huge crowded beer hall with a brass band, people drinking giant mugs of beer, and majestic churches. And, naturally, marvelous bakeries!

We had a light lunch at a nearby Ratskeller. I had Hungarian goulasch soup and Claire had a fish soup. We washed this down with Munich beer.

After a nap, we set out to find our way to the von Rad's by subway from Marienplatz station, carrying with us a box of German "pralines" (chocolate candies). We figured out the trains and were met by Michael and his son, Tobias, who spoke no English.

Michael drove us to his home. He said he had to have it built at great expense, indebting himself for life, because he could not find a suitable place to rent for a family of six. We met his wife, Rose, and children, Uta 15, Korinna 14, Tobias 11, and the baby boy, Sander. The children were beautiful and blond. The meal was cold meat cuts, cheeses, and salad with lettuce, tomatoes, and mushrooms. Before the meal Tobias, with whom I talked in German in my stumbling fashion, brought me a handful of precious strawberries from his own garden. His sister, Korinna, said he thought his strawberries were the best. They were small and, indeed, sweet and delicious.

After this pleasant family meal, with the baby in a high chair spilling something only once, Michael showed us around the new house, a three-story affair--typical European style. It would take pages to describe it.

We chatted over white wine after dinner, on professional and social matters. Claire and I got a bit intoxicated. But we found our way back, via the S-6, to our hotel.

September 17, 1985

At breakfast we again met the couple from New Jersey, John and Joyce Andrews; he was a director of marketing for an international industrial vacuum-cleaning-unit company. She, a mother of two, cuisiniere and vegetable gardener. Both, were on a vacation of 10 days. They gave us a printed summary of museums in Munich. Claire and I went to the New Pinakotkek where we saw an outstanding group of impressionist and pre-impressionist paintings. We had lunch there, too, and enjoyed local soups and, yes, beer. The waiter was a computer science student, who was openly adversely critical of Germany's place in the computer science competition.

Then we walked to the Residenzmuseum where we saw a huge collection of the rooms, clothing, paintings, porcelains, silver and bronze-gold dinner services, jewelry and so forth of the leaders and royalty of past history. We walked towards our hotel through a bustling traffic of autos and people, all on cobblestones. We sat down and had some refreshing drinks at an outdoor cafe in the midst of Theatinerstrasse, which is closed off to automobiles. We saw two bicyclists being given arrest tickets by the police for riding their bicycles rather than walking them through this great shopping center and parade of people looking at other people and at store windows.

We met Claudia Walther and her man, Vitus, a handsome bearded and balding chap, a Bavarian. She must be in her early fifties. He is 11 years younger. She is divorced and has a daughter, age 21, who is a radio announcer. He is divorced, too. Claudia said in front of us that Vitus' ex-wife couldn' t be trusted, but she could. Vitus spoke English about as well as I spoke German, maybe better. Claudia said his German was Bavarian German, different from hers, and that the Bavarians are slow-thinkers. They took us to a Bavarian restaurant and ordered Bavarian dinners for us. A man with a fine bold baritone voice played the accordian and sang Bavarian and American songs. A group of Americans came in and had dinner and joined the singer in American songs, such as, San Francisco, New York-New York, and so forth.

The beer consumed was sizeable, but Claire and I set limits on ourselves. Considering the probable income level of our host and hostess, I paid the food and drink bill. They protested feebly. They walked us back to our hotel, and we chatted.

SEPTEMBER 18, 1985

Today we knew we were free to plan to do whatever we wanted and meet no one.

Claire was planning to purchase a jacket that had captured her heart after extensive shopping. I accompanied her to the square (Marienplatz) where the store--Benetton--was located and watched all the people milling around. Tourists in smaller groups around a tour leader, native shoppers, workmen pulling up flat stones for some unknown reason. I took some photos.

Then Claire came out of the store and said they took no credit cards, and this stymied her intention to buy this marvelous jacket for I had agreed to provide some of the funds for the purchase. She was, obviously disappointed.

We spent a couple of hours shopping at department stores that took credit cards. They had a very wide selection of jackets and women's clothes. I enjoyed helping Claire find what she wanted, looking at the wide variety of clothes and prices, the attractive women, even the mannikins. Very few men were helping women at this enterprise. Claire, naturally, had ideas of her own on what she wanted, though many of the jackets looked good to me on her. I think she is on the conservative side. Also, she said she was thinking of what clothes she had at home that would match a prospective jacket. Anyway, she decided not to buy anything.

We ate lunch in a beautiful beer garden off the main street, which was bustling with crowds of people.

The waiter, a nice looking, young bearded man, spoke no English and was surly when Claire spoke to him in English. Claire ordered a sausage dish with mustard, and it was delicious. I ordered fish and the fish--something like a trout--was terrible. The waiter looked sad when I told him the fish was bad (schlect), but he charged us anyway. I did not care. The atmosphere was great.

After this lunch, Claire decided to buy the jacket she really wanted at Benetton's though she would have to pay German cash for it. Of course, I had to come to the rescue. We made a deal that if the sale of my portion of Specialty Medical Labs to Charter Hospitals went through, I would foot the cost of the jacket; otherwise, Claire owed me whatever I loaned her on the purchase.

I noticed Claire was jubilant after her purchase for 269 marks. Now we visited another museum, the Volkerkundemuseum, on 42 Maximilianstrasse. I especially liked the African Art exhibit there.

The Ethiopian art was concrete and primitive. The Phillipine art had some merit.

We returned to our hotel, took naps, and then went to the fine French-style restaurant La Bouillabaisse, in our Hotel. I had an exquisite lobster soup and Claire had a fine mushroom soup. Claire had a tender veal dish, and I had a truly fresh turbot--both entrees were in the French cuisine style and quite tasty. We each had desserts: Claire had plums in an aspic gel with a sauce and I had fresh fruit (kiwis, peaches, bananas, etc. sliced) in a wine sauce topped with whipped cream. All of this was accompanied by a bottle of French medium dry white wine. This was our last supper together, and we immersed ourselves in the ambience, food flavors, and good conversation.

SEPTEMBER 19, 1985

Though Claire set her electronic alarm clock for 5:15 a.m., and I asked the hotel clerk to give us a wake-up all at 5:15 a.m. so Claire could make her 7:15 a.m. Lufthansa flight out of Munich to Frankfurt so as to catch her 9:15 a.m. Condor Chart flight to Los Angeles, we both were awakened earlier by our internal clocks. We arrived at the Munich Flughaven early by taxi, purchased Claire's flight ticket to Frankfurt, sent two of her pieces of luggage straight through to Los Angeles, and relaxed with a cup of coffee with milk. I saw Claire go through the passenger checkpoint for her flight; she got into the wrong aisle--one for males--and a gentleman with an automatic rifle spoke to her in German to get into the aisle for females while suspiciously eyeing me standing nearby watching her. I told her in English to get into the other aisle, and she did so, and I watched her put her three handbags through the x-ray machine and I saw a women searching her body. Then off she went, while the chap with the beep gun kept a nervous eye on me. I retreated gracefully, hailed a taxi, and returned to my hotel. The return taxi fare was 19 marks and I gave the driver 40 marks. He said, without hesitation "That's too much," and he gave me back 20 marks. I gave him some loose change saying, "There's something for you honestly." The taxi ride to the Munich Flughaven had cost 30.80 marks (probably because there were two passengers), and I had given that driver 40 marks, and he had given me back the difference. As I write this, I can't tell whether I was perseverating, based on the taxi fare I paid going to the airport, or whether I was unnerved by the airport security officer with his machine gun or whether I was sad to see Claire go. Probably all of the above.

I went to the Deutsches Museum which exhibits scientific and technical developments and historical objects. There were many people there especially younger ones (in their teens and twenties). The exhibits were reminiscent of what one sees in the Museum of Science and Industry in Chicago and the Smithsonian Institute in Washington, D.C. One disadvantage for me, which I fully anticipated, was that all written explanations were in German. I looked up about 20 words in my little German dictionary, some of which were not in it--not a rare event. I loved the airplanes and took a picture of the three-winged Fokker and a cross-section of a wide-bodied plane similar to a DC 1011. The train display was really interesting, and I thought how Hampton would love it. How oil and gas wells are drilled, and how oil is refined was good to see. I walked around until my feet were tired and then walked outside and sat down to watch a clever water fountain in which water filled oblong tubs that eventually dumped the water into another such tub that, when filled, turned and dumped out its water. While bserving and pondering this clever affair, I overheard a late middle-aged dumpy and unattractive American couple sitting nearby arguing with each other about the discomfort of their plane flight and about the inconveniences they were encountering in Germany. I wanted momentarily to be closer so I could overhear them better, but I reminded myself I was off-duty and didn' t have to fathom their problems.

The day was sunny and warmer than I had previously experienced in Germany. I had a light sweater and a suit coat, and I was uncomfortably warm and wondered whether Italy would be like that.

When I got back to my hotel via taxi, the cab driver and I chatting with each other all the way in his bad English and I in my poor Germany, 10 Falkenturnstrasse was clogged up by a dump trunk. So I hopped out of the taxi, so the cab driver could back up on this narrow one-way street (einbahnstasse).

The time was early afternoon. So I finished reading my book on artificial intelligence and fifth generation computers (E.A. Feigenbaum, and P. McCorduck, *The Fifth Generation.* New York: New American Library, 1984), which is a very repetitious book composed of many chapters most of which say precisely what was said in a half-dozen previous chapters. Still, it was capable of putting me in the mood to write my own monograph on "The Computerization of the Content Analysis of Natural Language," when I get to Bellagio, Italy.

While so engaged, Claudia telephoned to tell me it was possible to phone "collect" to the USA, by first dialing "0010." That puzzled me because my German friends in Freiburg and Hamburg said it was difficult or impossible to do so. I may try it.

I also reread my paper on "The Emotional Impact of Mastectomy," and I checked the slides that go with it so I could perform smoothly tomorrow at the Stadtisches Krankenhaus Munchen-Bogenhausen-Abteilung fur, Psychosomatische Medizin und Psychotherapie. I found the paper to be of a high standard, though it reported what one might have guessed, proving the findings in elegant and sophisticated research design and statistics.

For a change in diet and atmosphere I decided to eat at Harry's New York Bar that was just a few buildings down the Falkenturnstrasse from my Hotel. The atmosphere seemed more European than American. It was a small bar with about six small tables in the room. It had a modest sized bar with bar stools. The bartender spoke English with a German accent. I ordered a beer and asked for a menu. In about eight minutes, I got my beer and the menu. English was being spoken by most of the few people sitting around. Two guys, each alone, one sitting at the bar and the other sitting at a table, eyed me sullenly and continuously. They were odd-looking, I thought they might be both curious and maybe lonely. I returned their dour looking with only brief glances, ordered a Harry's specialty, a steak sandwich, and read the copy of the USA Today newspaper I had just bought over at the Vierjahreszeiten Hotel. In about 10 minutes the sandwich arrived. The steak was about 7/16 of an inch thick and the size of two American silver dollars, on a 3/8 inch slice of gravy-soaked bread. On the plate was a large serving of cole slaw on a piece of crisp lettuce. In addition I was served a small dish containing more lettuce topped with a tomato sauce containing onions. So this was Harry's steak sandwich. I had read about this sandwich, especially in American detective stories. The appearance of this sandwich did not coincide at all with what I had fantasied. But I put it to further tests--the cutting and taste tests. It barely passed the cutting test, for it was slightly firmer meat than my imagination anticipated. However, it did pass the taste test. It certainly should have because it was helped considerably by my appetite, for I had skipped eating lunch. I cleaned up every bit of steak and available piece of slaw and salad.

When I got back to the hotel there was a message from Michael von Rad that he would pick me up tomorrow at 10:45 a.m. in front of the Hotel Vierjahreszeiten on Maximilianstrasse.

SEPTEMBER 20, 1985

I was ready and waiting 15 minutes early for Michael von Rad to pick me up in front of the Hotel Vierjahreszeiten. I walked up and down the block in front of it to get some exercise and to tranquilize myself. Michael--in the already heavy traffic--came 10 minutes early in his Peugot. Was this an example of two over-punctual Germans, anticipating each other's moves? He drove to his hospital, a new 1000-bed facility. It was only one year old, and I found it be truly magnificent. The doctors ' offices, the patients' rooms, and patients eating places, recreational facilities, diagnostic facilities, everything was truly on a grand, artistic, and well-planned basis. I asked Michael who built the hospital and how much did it cost. He said it was built by the City of Munich, and it cost 150,000,000 marks to construct. I asked him did all the patients have insurance, and he said that in Germany all people have to have health insurance.

His own Psychosomatic Division has a 60-bed inpatient unit. There is a 40-bed psychosomatic subdivision and a 20-bed somatopsychic subdivision. At present he has no chronic psychotic psychiatric patients who have developed medical or surgical disorders. Such patients are cared for by the Psychiatric Division of the University of Munich. If he were asked to accept such patients, he would do so; for he could imagine that such patients might need special and expert management. He has a staff of 13.5; they could all be physicians, but he has used two of these positions to hire medical psychologists. He has another three psychologists on his staff.

I have not seen any hospital facilities, public or private, quite so elegant and well conceived for patient care as the Stadtisches Krankenhaus Munchen-Bogenhausen. My presentation on the "Emotional Impact of Mastectomy" began at 11:30 a.m. and was concluded at 1:00 p.m. The audience of about 25 people was intelligent and appreciative. Michael gave my professional background and affiliations in German--as had Uwe Koch, in Freiburg and Adolph Meyer in Hamburg. And he gave a summary presentation, in German, of the Gottschalk- Gleser Verbal Content Analysis Measures, which helped my presentation a great deal, for some of the members of the audience were not familiar with this measurement method .

He invited me to lunch at the hospital cafeteria. There was a standard meal dished out in the cafeteria (like at Michael Reese Hospital in Chicago): a main course of spaghetti with a sauce of tomatoes, ground meat, and mushrooms (the portions filled the whole dinner plate), another plate of a big salad, a dessert (something that looked like yogurt, and tasted very good, but Michael said it was schmeerkase). I asked for a half-portion of the spaghetti dish, which I thought was good.

During the meal I talked to some of Michael's staff. Around me were some women medical internists who, also, had another degree, such as, in psychology or psychiatry. These women happened to speak excellent English and they had been to the USA several times. One women I met was Dr. Sell-Schott, who is Chief of Psychosomatic Medicine in a Cancer Treatment Institute (Michael said she was the "Jimmie Holland" of West Germany; Jimmie Holland is a psychiatrist friend of mine who is Chief of Psychiatry at the Sloan-Kettering Institute in New York City). Dr. Sell-Schott says she plans to use the Gottschalk-Gleser scales in her next cancer research study.

Michael and I spent some time in the early afternoon discussing professional matters. Then he said his wife, Rose, said the von Rad family should go to the USA in March--April 1986 because the girls, especially the oldest, were maybe getting to the upper age limit when they would want to do something as a family. He added that if his wife volunteered such, he would certainly want to go. Besides California, he likes the deserts of Arizona and New Mexico, and he wondered whether they might be attractive at this time. I told him they might be flowering then and that should he bring his family to the USA, we would facilitate his trip. Michael paid me 400 marks cash for my lecture and conference, apologizing how small the amount was. I told him that was as much or more than we paid visiting professors and that academicians are supposed to work for love not money.

After making my farewells to Michael, I decided to spend the rest of the afternoon walking and revisiting, especially, Marienplatz. There were more people than ever there. Musicians and actors were attracting audiences every 50-100 feet. There was a string trio, a solo clarinetist, a flutist and bassoonist, an accordionist, a single violinist, and on-and-on. There was, even, a guy who did balancing acts on a unicycle and a high ladder while juggling. He turned out to be from New Orleans, LA! I got thirsty walking around. And it was warm. I got thirstier walking into an outdoor market where lots of people were standing or sitting while drinking beer. I decided not to drink beer but to walk to a McDonald' s and get a milkshake. There was a long line and when I got to my turn the girl said they were out of milkshakes. So I got a coke instead.

Returning to my hotel, I was there when Helen phoned, and we had a good talk. Also, Andres phoned, and I said I had decided not to go to Berlin but to head for Innsbruck, Austria and, then, to Italy. He told me he had been approved for a month's vacation and was coming to the USA from December 14, 1985 to January 14, 1986.

I decided to go to the Bouillabaisse Restaurant in my hotel for my last night in Munich. I am not disappointed I did so. I had bouillabaisse, served with croutons and a hot sauce that could be used to the amount one wanted. It was more than acceptable. Then I had a desert of strawberry and pistachio ices topped with whipped cream. Everyone around me spoke only German. A pretty girl that looked and acted just like my daughter Louise sat diagonally facing me at another table. Mental telepathy did not work on her. Very near me sat a big thirty-fivish German man, facing a small, young woman, and he shot a continual aggressive stream of speech at this woman, but periodically she would come back at him, in a softer but assertive voice and he would reply, Ja, ja, ja, O.k. or "Nein, nein, nein, nein" I could only catch some of the words, like "the English, psychology, chemicals," and so forth, all in German. I could, unfortunately, never catch enough to make a mystery, spy thriller, or adulterous relationship out of this twosome.

Then I climbed into bed, eagerly looking forward to my drive to Innsbruck, Austria tomorrow, where I had been once before in my life.

SEPTEMBER 21, 1985

I remember on awakening three topics I failed to make journal notes on yesterday.

(1) I told Michael von Rad that at UCIMC we were considering developing a small Psychiatric Medicine Unit of about 15 beds in the General Hospital portion of UCIMC and

we would not call it a Psychosomatic Unit because that name would not include somatopsychic and other types of patients we see on our Psychiatric Consultation and Liaison Division. He said that in Germany the term "psychosomatische" is the medically acceptable term for all activities that his service does and "psychiatrische" is not.

(2) My secretary, Linda, said Carolyn Winget would score verbal samples for me for a price that and that I will likely get $5,000 from the MacArthur Foundation to do the study on emotional factors in relatives of schizophrenics that predispose to relapse of the schizophrenic. I intend to write Caroline to score conservatively the speech samples we send her.

(3) Oh yes, and one more topic I learned from Linda, via Helen yesterday, was that my novel will not be completed by the printer until October 1, 1985. Too bad, Helen will not be able to bring me a final printed copy on September 26.

Well, I got off from Munich about 8:30 a.m. after settling my hotel bill and retrieving my rental Opel Kadette. I followed Michael's instructions and kept looking for a blue sign indicating the autobahn to Salzburg. I seemed to be going long distances in the City, but his advice was valid. I got on the autobahn to Salzburg and found the turnoff to Innsbruck. Suddenly the traffic slowed to a creep. Then a helicopter came over my car and landed a small distance ahead in the lanes going in the opposite direction. I figured it was an accident, and I was right. I snapped a photo of it as I passed by.

Behind that accident the traffic was blocked for miles.

I pushed along to Innsbruck, going about 100-130 km/hr. As Michael had said, this route to Innsbruck is in a valley with the mountains beginning to rise on both sides. I took a photo from my driver's seat. When I got to Innsbruck, it was early, about 11:30 a.m. I spoke to an information guide (he spoke English), and he said if I wanted to drive another 2.5-3.0 hours, it would be easy to make St. Moritz, and he assured me all the passes were clear. I decided to go for it--St. Moritz, here I come. I was exhilarated driving again, though I missed Claire's companionship. Besides, I was feeling psychologically crippled with my German, and I was longing to speak French again.

The drive to St. Moritz was marvelous from the scenery point of view. I could imagine how Helen, Claire, and all the other members of my family would rave about it. Not better than the Western part of the USA, but different.

I was awed and scared a bit by a few of the European drivers passing me and others at mountain turns going uphill or downhill. I went through Austrian customs, and, then, through Italian Swiss customs, having only to show my American passport. I got to St. Moritz and it was on a lake surrounded by some snow-capped mountains. I did not know where to look for a hotel. One section in which I found myself, was near the lake; the buildings and hotels were of the high-rise type. That did not fit with my concept of St. Moritz. I noted that the signs were all in Italian or German, and my car radio stations were, also, only in Italian or German. No French!

Well, I persevered and followed the German signs reading St. Moritz Dorf instead of St. Moritz Bad and found the older part of St. Moritz, parked and tried to speak to some people. Most of them spoke Italian and nothing else. I did find a German-speaking woman, who also spoke Schweizer-Deutsch (Swiss-German). The car radio had some Swiss-German stations. The German speaking lady said the Hotel Post was a good one and pointed vaguely in the direction I should go. I did find it, through winding, ascending, and narrow streets. I kept on looking some more and found a small hotel that pleased me more. They did not have a single room--which went for 60 Fr.--but had a double, which went for 100 Fr and they would let me have it for 75 Fr. I had Austrian schillings, Italian lira, American dollars, German marks, and this hotel, the Hotel Eden Garni St. Moritz, did not accept any credit cards. I had only a vague idea of the exchange rate for Swiss francs. I found out that there were about 2.30 Swiss francs to an American dollar. The desk clerk, a pretty blond girl, said they would accept German marks. I took the room; it was very neat and roomy with a nice private bath.

I took a quick 25-minute nap and ventured out. I walked about 1.5 miles downhill to the railroad station, the only place I could change money on Saturday. I got Swiss francs for my Austrian money and for a 100 mark German note.

I walked some more back uphill. I ran into a big brass band of clowns serenading a couple (one of them a part-owner of a hotel and the other the hired director) getting married. The bride and groom and wedding guests had 6 horse-drawn carriages to haul them around St. Moritz. The horses had tiny tinkling bells on them. I got a photo of the clown band playing.

I ate a dinner of a ham and cheese sandwich topped by a fried egg washed down with a bottle of dark beer. The sandwich was built like I have never seen or had. The toast was buried under a large amount of warm Gruyere cheese, covered with a slice of ham and a fried egg, sunny-side up. It was good and, certainly, filled me up.

I returned to my room, took a soaking hot bath, and got into one of the double beds with those fully, air-filled covers--a feather bed cover. I never ate so much Gruyere cheese at one sitting.

I guess I am going to have to get used to not hearing much French or English on the streets of St. Moritz. The desk clerks, though, all speak English or French--at least the two I have encountered at the Hotel Eden Garni.

September 22, 1985

On awakening a little before 7:00 a.m., I got to thinking it might be a good idea to call Helen now--instead of waiting until the evening on European time--and let her know where I was. I had told her I was driving only as far as Innsbruck, Austria. I probably woke up the poor dear woman for the phone rang four times before she picked it up. Her time was 10:00 p.m. She told me that Ray was selling his business, which would be good for both Ray and Claire and would get Helen and I off the hook of guaranteeing Ray's loans.

I learned at breakfast-time that "Garni" in the hotel name meant bed and breakfast. The breakfast served, without extra charge, at the Hotel Eden was quite elegant for my tastes. It included the usual things that appear in a so-called "continental" breakfast, coffee, tea, or milk, rolls, butter, and jams. The three rolls I was provided were the best ever: two small, round, fresh-baked, crisp-crusted buns and one light, flaky croissant. In addition, there was a loaf of brown bread from which I would help myself, but did not. And a long tart stuffed with fruit-apples--from which I took a 1.5 inch slice. Moreover, there was a clear plastic-covered plate that had Swiss cheese slices and packages of assorted ground meats, such as "schinkenkase." I took only one of the cheese slices. Everything tasted good. That was a big breakfast!

On the advice of the hotel proprietor I drove over to the Heilingbadhaus to listen to an outdoor concert at 10:30 a.m. I waited around and the concert never took place. That was the second time I had gone to hear a free outdoor concert and it did not occur--the first time was in Gottingen. I asked a woman in the Kurgarden whether the concert was going to take place. She shook her head and said she spoke only Italian, and pointed to another woman who spoke a little German. The second woman indicated she did not know about a concert that morning and pointed to another nearby couple. I had a sheet of paper that was at my hotel breakfast table telling all the events of the day and, in clear German, detailing the place and time of the music concert. This third couple spoke some German and the lady of the couple knew a few words of English. She looked at my sheet of paper and acknowledged there should be a concert. She went off the scene with my paper, while I exchanged a few more words with her husband. He had a sense of humor, for he said in German, maybe the concert was called off because of the weather. But the sky was blue and the weather was warm. We both laughed, and he winked. His lady came back and announced that there was supposed to be concert, but the concert players must have taken the week off. We all laughed.

I decided to drive up to one of the mountain passes the hotel proprietor had suggested. He said I could either take the train or drive to it, if I had an auto. I drove.

It did not take long to get to it. On the way I took some photos of snow-covered mountains. The mountain pass I went to was "Passo del Bernina." The elevation was 2330 meters. The mountains were impressive, and there were three small lakes just below us; two were rather clear and one was milky blue. I did not find out how come.

Next, I came back to St. Moritz, disposed of my coat and sweater at my hotel because it was getting warm. And I drove up the mountain behind St. Moritz Dorf (town) and my hotel. The road got narrower and narrower. At one stretch it had to be one car at a time. But I encountered no car coming down. My goal was to reach a large building perched high up on the mountainside. When I got there I could see it was a large, old, fine hotel that was closed. A few other people with cars were parked in front of it--it had the name "Chaperella" on it--and the people were looking at or taking pictures of the magnificent view. I parked and looked and photographed. I could see a funiculaire coming up the mountainside to the far side this hotel. I walked over towards it, and on inquiry a man explained the lane for this vehicle was being extended to the mountaintop and would be completed by December. I deduced that was probably why the big Hotel Chaperella was closed now, and this mountainside conveyance would facilitate coming to the hotel a safer way than by the narrow road I had traversed and could, furthermore, provide access for skiers to the skiing sites higher up.

I still had a lot of energy. So I left my car parked there, and I walked about two miles up a narrow road. I came across a small outdoor restaurant serving drinks and food on a balcony overlooking the valley, had a beer and, though I was not very hungry after my huge breakfast, got a bowl of goulasch soup served with bread. I had a very leisurely lunch, not hearing any English, but plenty of German and Italian.

Oh yes, people had their dogs along--as in most of Europe--and there was a dog fight or near fight. The masters of the dogs persisted in trying to have the dogs make friends, but one of the dogs could not understand what its master was trying to say. That reminded me that one of my fellow hotel guests had a dog about the size of a St. Bernard but it was black and white. Was he charged for a double-room? I also noted, that the lovely breakfast room in my hotel had a sign in German saying that dogs had to be on a leash in there or could not be allowed entrance.

Anyway, I came back to my hotel to relax and read, having bought a Financial Times, published out of London. I have found the articles in it very clearly written, very scholarly, and quite enlightening. More important the Financial Times covers world news. I read the first clear account of the earthquake in Mexico City. What a mess! At least some of the high-rise earthquake-proof buildings survived. Shades of what could happen in California?

I also read in Newsweek an article about Elizabeth Taylor accompanied by a photo of her revealing her bosomy cleavage. The photo was taken at the Hotel Royal in Deauville, France, where there had recently been a film festival. That was the same hotel where Claire, George, and I had had drinks one fine afternoon!

I went out from the hotel about 6:00 p.m. for a long walk and explored most of the rest of St. Moritz. I really did not feel hungry. So I decided to skip supper. I found a store that had magazines and, surprisingly, a Time and Newsweek in English. I got a Newsweek.

Returning to my hotel, I spent a quiet evening devouring my Newsweek and some more of my Financial Times. This whole travel experience has made me realize how much time I spend looking at television, probably, much less time than other Americans. Take away that television-watching time and one has hours daily that are open for other kinds of living experiences. I am both a workaholic and a playaholic--I like to squeeze into my waking hours some kind of stimulating interesting, attention-holding, time-consuming activity.

SEPTEMBER 23, 1985

I prepared to drive on to Italy towards Bellagio and Lake Como. I had another fine breakfast at the Hotel Eden, paid my hotel bill, and pointed my Opel in the right direction towards Bellagio. I followed the road signs, now a narrowing two-lane black-topped road, navigating by a blue sign that pointed the way towards two passes. Which pass was I supposed to take? I had no detailed map of Italy, except a sketchy one in my Michelin Guide for Italy and an Automobile Club map. None of them designated any specific passes on the road I was taking. On one map I could see the name of a mountain area--Maloja--that was identical to one of the pass names on the blue sign. That must be the pass to take. So when the blue signs indicated the road to the two passes was diverging, I took the road to the left, towards the Maloja Pass, crossing my fingers, I drove gradually up, and then, over the Maloja Pass, and then I wound down, back and forth, for many miles into a valley. I drove through many little villages that looked very old. The roofs of the houses were made of flat stones and the streets were so narrow at places only one car could pass. I finally came to the Swiss-Italian border. The Swiss customs waved me through. The Italian customs wanted to see my passport. "Americana" he said as he studied it. "Si," I said, using my big Italian vocabulary.

Then he asked me something I could not, initially, understand, though I barely caught the word "whiskey." He repeated his question two times, and I discerned the words "whiskey" and "sigaretta." I quickly got the message and replied, with my best Italian accent. "No." And he waved me on. I, in turn, asked him a question, pointing straight ahead--"Bellagio?" He gave no sign of recognition. "Como, Como?" I persisted. "Si, Como," he nodded and pointed ahead. I sighed in relief. Well, then, I drove and drove, often through many tunnels, in a beautiful valley, mountains on either side, and once in a while with a lake on one side of me or the other, which I supposed and hoped might be Lake Como but was not. I followed the blue signs pointing to Milano. Finally, I got to a long, long lake that had to be Lake Como. But I never got to Bellagio. I stopped in one of the larger lakeside towns and asked a man,

"Bellagio?" and pointed to my map. He scrutinized it, and speaking only Italian, he indicated I should drive to Lecco and turn to the right; Bellagio was on the tip of a promontory that jutted out into Lake Como. I drove along a lakeside road, feasting on beautiful scenery, for about an hour and arrived at Bellagio. By this time, around noontime, I had formulated a plan to locate the Villa Serbelloni where the Rockefeller Study Center was, tell them I had driven to Bellagio and I knew I had arrived one day early, and could they help me find a hotel to stay in? Of course, I was hoping they would, somehow, find accommodations for me, even though they had said when I phoned them from my Munich Hotel that I should not arrive until the early afternoon of September 24 because my accommodations at the Rockefeller Study Center were occupied up to that time.

I drove into Bellagio, finally, and somehow located the Grand Hotel--Villa~Serbelloni. It was an attractive, large, old building on the lake, and stylish-looking people were sitting here and there. I found a desk clerk and asked "Rockefeller Study Center?" He shook his head negatively and said it was up on top the hill and waved his hand ambiguously in some direction. It was, also, called "Villa Serbelloni," he explained.

I will not describe how I found the specific Villa Serbelloni for which I was looking--it would take too many pages. The only entrance by auto is via a large wrought iron gate that opens automatically by someone operating it from a distant location inside a 50-acre estate, if you can convince someone inside through a telephone at the gate you should be allowed entrance. I gained entrance by talking to a woman on the phone, identifying myself and telling her my rehearsed story. She told me that the people who had occupied my rooms had departed. I drove my Opel up a long hill to a large, stately, yellow building and parked in a parking lot. I noticed three people standing outside the front door waiting for me. They introduced themselves: a Mr. and Mrs. McKelvey--who were temporarily substituting for a Mrs. Ardovini, the regular hostess, who had suffered a fall and Mr. Roberto Celli, the Chief Administrator, who was away--and a porter, in a uniform, to carry my luggage.

I was taken by Mrs. McKelvey to my room, number 5, which was very large and elegant, in a 17th-18th century style, with an entrance way, a private bath, two large closets, a private study, and a magnificent overview of Lake Como. She, also, gave me a set of papers to read, pointing out one in particular that, she said, described the house rules for guests ("A Guide for Resident guests"). She added that tea and coffee were being served, and if I wanted some, I should come now and I could meet some of the guests.

It was now early afternoon, and I was tired of driving and a bit hungry. So I went along with her, barely glancing at the 18th century decor, including tapestries and furnishings, as we walked down a long hallway to a room, where about 10 people were chatting and having tea.

While I sipped on some cafe au lait sweetened with sugar, to raise my blood glucose, she introduced me to fellow beneficiaries of the Rockefeller Foundation .

I am not going to relate in this journal the pleasure and awe I experienced the afternoon and evening of September 23, 1985 being at the Villa Serbelloni, the rejuvenation I had walking down the very long path to Lake Como and taking a swim, meeting more people at 7:00 p.m. for apéritifs and sitting down at 7:30 p.m for a rather formal gourmet dinner (jacket and tie required for the gentlemen). Nor will I elaborate on the delight I experienced meeting and talking to the other guests, my pleasure certainly being enhanced by my recent relative lack of companionship on this journey since Claire's departure. My appetite was whetted for human conversation and exchange of ideas. Clearly, there would be ample opportunity for such exchanges at the Villa Serbelloni as well as a good occasion to do all the writing I wanted to do and maintain as much privacy as I required. I retired happy and fulfilled, anticipating how much satisfaction Helen would have being at this place when she would arrive by Alitalia Airlines in Milan around 2:35 p.m. September 26, 1985.

September 24, 1985

This is a good point at which to end this journal, having arrived at the destination that led me to come to Europe at this time. I can see, this morning, that life at the Rockefeller Study and Conference Center, Villa Serbelloni, Bellagio, Italy, is going to lead through much different pathways than were encountered in the travels through France and Germany with Claire. Perhaps another journal or, certainly, some kind of accounts of the experiences at Villa Serbelloni will unfold from Helen or from my viewpoint. Let us wait and see.

American College of Neuropsychopharmacology

December 1996

Interviewed by: Dr. William E. Bunney Jr. (WB)

WB: I am Dr. William Bunney, Professor of Psychiatry and Human Behavior, University of California at Irvine. I am interviewing, today, Professor Louis A. Gottschalk, who is also Professor of Psychiatry at the University of California, Irvine, and the Founding Chairman of the Department of Psychiatry and Human Behavior (1967-1978) at the University of California, Irvine. He is one of the premier neuropsychopharmacologists in our field. And, Louis, I would like to ask you, can you tell us a little bit about your training?

LG: Yes. Well, I was born in St. Louis, Missouri, and I went to university at Washington University in St. Louis, Missouri. I attended undergraduate school there. As I reflect on it now, I had the good fortune of having some very inspiring scientific educators, as an undergraduate. And, then, I went to the Washington University Medical School. And there, I didn't realize it at the time, I was being programmed by a number of Nobel Prize laureates. At Washington University undergraduate school, there was Arthur Holly Compton, a Nobel Prize winning physicist. At the Medical School, I was a student under Carl and Gertie Cory, Nobel Prize biochemists, and James Erlanger, a Nobel Prize winning physiologist. And I didn't know it, but I just seemed naturally to be molded and shaped into doing a lot of research. Beginning as a medical student, I had a position working as a research assistant (funded by the Josiah Macy Foundation) under some famous professors in the Department of Neuropsychiatry. There was David Rioch, whom I believe you know. The Neuropsychiatry Department was headed by John C. Whitehorn, who, already back in those times, had a neurobiochemical view of the etiology and pathogenesis of neuropsychiatric illnesses. And another interesting person in that Department was the man that did the first frontal ablation experiments in subhuman animals; his name was Carlyle Jacobson, Ph.D.; he did these studies while he was still at Yale University. In any case, that's where I got my medical school training, and I did an internship in straight medicine at Washington University, Barnes Hospital. And, in those days, it may happen again, the Departments of Psychiatry and Neurology were together in one Department. And, so my residency was in Neurology and Psychiatry at Barnes and McMillan Hospitals at Washington University, St. Louis. And, then, I think around 1946, I had to go into the military service (it was during World War II), and I was invited to transfer from the U.S. Army (in which I was in the reserve corps during my internship and residency) to the United States Public Health Service USPHS). As a matter of fact, I had a couple of more years of accredited neuropsychiatric training while I was stationed at the United States Public Health Hospital in Fort Worth, Texas. This hospital, which was a so-called "narcotic" hospital (a 2000 bed hospital on 10,000 acres) had been transformed into a neuropsychiatric hospital to diagnose and care for neuropsychiatric casualties resulting from military service during World War II. I was one of many psychiatrists (from the USPHS and Navy) looking after these neuropsychiatrically disabled Navy and Marine Corps service people there. I had some more training in Chicago, Illinois, in Child Psychiatry at the Michael Reese Neuropsychiatric and Psychosomatic Center. There, I also ran the (EEG) Electroencephalography laboratory. In those days, in the late nineteen forties, it was still in style to get psychoanalytic training. I got that kind of training at the Chicago Institute for Psychoanalysis in child and adult psychoanalysis.

WB: You had some really impressive mentors along the way, people who were really giants in the field.

LG: I was lucky; I really was. In Chicago, I worked under Roy R. Grinker at Michael Reese and at the Institute for Psychoanalysis, I trained under Franz Alexander and Thomas French. I was lucky, and didn't realize it.

WB: What first got you interested in psychopharmacology?

LG: I was programmed very young, I think, actually, to do research and when psychoactive drugs came along, I was right in to neuropsychopharmacology, very interested to learn more about them. And, that was about when chlorpromazine came along in, probably 1957 or something like that. And, also, the advent of the benzodiazepines. And, what happened, I think was, after my training in Chicago, I went to the National Institute of Mental Health. I was, in fact, the first research psychiatrist at NIMH. It was probably in 1951, and, again, I encountered David Rioch who was Chief of Neuropsychiatry at Walter Reed Army Hospital. In Chicago, I had got ten interested in epilepsy and the trigger mechanisms of epilepsy in children. And I took a group of epileptic kids, who were on anticonvulsant drugs, and the anticonvulsant drugs were not being effective with regards to their epilepsy. I tried psychotherapy or play therapy with them or other types of therapy and, lo and behold, for many of them their seizures disappeared. And, I wrote and published about those findings. So, when I went to the National Institute of Mental Health, and I wondered what kind of research was I going to do here, I asked myself? Where is the area where there might be the most novel and productive ideas? I thought about that for a while, and I went to Walter Reed Hospital and I did find some more patients that had epileptiform paroxysms in their EEG's. I thought, well, maybe I can find out what happens if you just have these patients free-associate (this idea came to me because I had had this psychoanalytic training), while you are getting their EEG's. I selected patients who had paroxysms of abnormal EEG's and I found out, in some of those people, when they spoke about emotional things, they showed more such EEG paroxysms. At that point, it came to me that one of the most inexact areas in the field of psychiatry was dealing with interviews and the things that people said and the ways in which they said them. At that point, I decided, well, it would not be a bad idea to try to develop more objective ways of arriving at more measures of anxiety or hostility as well as how schizophrenic somebody is. That diagnostic achievement is generally accomplished through the neuropsychiatric interview and the content and form of language. So, it was there that I started to get into the measurement of neuropsychiatric states and traits from the content analysis of speech and verbal texts. And, when I left NIMH to become Research Professor of Psychiatry at the University of Cincinnati, some of the new drugs were being developed by the pharmaceutical industry and coming on the market. And I got into trying to decide how to measure the effects of psychoactive drugs. I actually got into some early clinical trials to determine whether or not a drug like diazapam (valium) or chlordiazepoxide (librium) might, indeed, be anti-anxiety agents. We did placebo-drug studies, and we got five-minute speech samples, which would measure, objectively, with a method I had developed whether or not subjects were less anxious when they were on the benzodiazepines, and these were the early psychopharmacological studies.

WB: How did you come up with this idea, the five-minute speech sample, because I know this was something you developed and expanded on very successfully?

LG: It was at this point, I can remember very clearly working at Walter Reed, interviewing patients, epileptic patients and non-epileptic patients who had abnormal paroxysms of EEG's. And then I reflected that there are very sensitive technologies for measuring, accurately, many neurobiological phenomena (using biochemical measures and physiological approaches, such as recording brain waves). But we have no very accurate means of measuring the magnitude of various psychobiological states. There is, of course, the diagnostic interview, and the neuropsychiatrically focused diagnostic interview, which requires a verbal dialogue. And, at that point, I decided, hey, this is it! This could be a tough research field, but why not get into this research area? I had, also, been an English major, as well as a biology and chemistry major at undergraduate school. And that background facilitated my getting into the measurement of neuropsycho- biological dimensions. I thought it would certainly have some use if a reliable and valid testing procedure could be developed. The challenge was that the development of such a measurement procedure would have to go through many stages.

I should, here, give some acknowledgment to a person I met at the University of Cincinnati---Goldine C. Gleser. She had a a doctorate degree, a Ph.D., and had specialized in measurement psychology. She had been a math major. She helped me, in some aspect, on the statistical side of doing some of the problems to be solved in developing a measurement tool for detecting and assessing the magnitude of various psychobiological states.

I do not think that I should get into more detail about statistical problems, but these will come up again, for I can see that the research areas that I have gotten into, especially with drugs and other biochemical factors in neuropsychiatric illness, has followed me. In any case, I have continued to persist in working in the content analysis of language and have developed a computerized method of doing this, because I, sincerely, believe that in time, instead of psychiatric interviews or the use of various adjective check lists or other methods of measuring the magnitude of various psychological and psychiatric states, I think we will be using the computer, and we will, actually, use, I think, voice recognition. I am working on that now, but, in any case, (I've digressed a bit), but that's....

WB: No, no, but Doc, I think it's one of the central issues that you've made a major contribution with this. And, if I understand, this has to do with diagnosis, has to do with diagnosis of emotions and has been used to follow behavioral change after medications. Is this correct? Are all these relevant?

LG: Absolutely right. And, I have kept following those ideas. As I think about it now, I do recall that what inspired me, some of the people at Washington University Medical School, James Bishop, a neurophysiologist, David Rioch, those fine neuroscientists, the way they thought, and they way pursued things, I think just got transferred and internalized in me. But, in any case, with regards to psychiatric drugs, I did get involved after a while in looking at the blood levels of and the pharmacokinetics of psychoactive drugs, such as the benzodiazepines.

WB: This was in Cincinnati?

LG: This was in Cincinnati. And, I found that, yes, if you had too low a blood level, you did not get any definite antianxiety effect, but over a blood level of a certain level, there was this significant correlation between the anxiety scores, that is, a reduction in anxiety scores derived from my Content Analysis Scales and the blood level of the benzodiazepine as well as the half life of the benzodiazepine. I, also, found that some of the benzodiazepines produce some cognitive impairment, or at least, impairment of memory, recent memory, and that's related to blood levels. And, from that, I got into looking at the effects of some of the major tranquilizers on schizophrenia, like thioridazine and mesoridazine. I found that, yes, the blood levels of those drugs, up to a certain extent with some schizophrenic patients, did correlate positively with an improvement. There was about a third of those schizophrenic patients that did not have a very favorable response to those major tranquilizers, but two-thirds did.

WB: Now, your Content Analysis Scales have had international acceptance, as I understand it.

LG: Yes, one might expect they would. The German neuroscientists got interested in that sort of methodological approach and they have borrowed and used my ideas. They published a number of books using my content analysis methodology. The Chairman of the Department of Psychiatry in Hamburg, Germany, told me that he and his colleagues got a $1,000,000.00 research grant from the German government to test and apply our content analysis methodology to their neuropsychiatric research. And, since then, their studes have been published. The procedure has been published in Spanish (especially in Chile), in Norway, Poland, Australia, Italy, the Netherlands, Germany, and in many different languages. And people have asked us, lately, and from other countries, have we got a computer program in their language to do this? Which is rather awesome that they would ask such a question, because computer programs are not readily transformed and adaptable to any and all languages. We are, currently, working on a computer program that will handle the Spanish language. Why select the Spanish language; because such a large percentage of the world's population speaks Spanish. But, yes, it has been found that the norms that we have in normal individuals, for anxiety and hostility, are not any different from the norms in Norway or Australia or in Germany. I suspect and think there's a difference in a country like Poland. I have had a visiting professor that's lived there and is coming to visit us again, and she found that, I am not surprised, having suffered the ravages of war, the norms there for anxiety run a little bit higher than the American's norms. But, yes, there's been a good deal of international interest in our methodology.

WB: It is translatable, internationally, is the issue.

LG: Yes, it is, but not the computer program.

WB: That's a major effort, in itself, to translate that. Are there specific hypotheses that you've tested in some of this work, one way of thinking about it?

LG: Yes. Well, some hypotheses. I think an obvious one was the blood levels of a drug should be related to the clinical effect. That is, within certain parameters, such is true. But if the blood level is too low, we have found out the drug is not going to have an effect. Also, you can give too large a drug dose, and we did find that above a certain blood level produces no more favorable clinical effect. That's for immediate effect of the drug. And there was another hypothesis that hasn't really got ten much attention and I notice it has not had much effect yet, perhaps, in neuropsychopharmacology at these meetings or other meetings. That is, we got interested in the finding that thioridazine in some people or mesoridazine in some people, produce adverse cardiovascular effects, cardiac irregularities. And at the time we were studying those phenomena and getting electrocardiographic measurements and drug blood levels on patients, we got the idea, let us find out whether there are any differences in the psychoactive drug metabolites of the people that get these cardiac irregularities. And lo and behold, we did discover that a metabolite that is not thought to be active psychoactively, it indeed, is not, namely, sulfaridizine, does have an adverse cardiovascular effect. And, that these individuals that had the cardiac irregularities had elevated sulfaridizine at that time. We were excited about that and published that finding, and we tried to get the drug companies to provide further financial support so we could study the biochemical basis for the adverse cardiovascular effect of sulfaridazine. But, under that circumstances, they were doing so well marketing the drug, that the drug company would not fund it. But, I mention it now because the whole area of abnormal effects, side-effects, I think, will be studied, perhaps, more and more. I think we are caught so much in the excitement about the favorable effects of drugs that the possibility that a drug's metabolites in everybody may be slightly different, except perhaps for identical twins, has not been focused on. And, we do metabolize these drugs slightly differently. And, those subtle drug-metabolite effects, sometimes, are cardinal and important and that fact can influence and obscure expected findings. I think that matter might become more and more important. It has not been followed up very much. So, that was one of the hypotheses that we had too, namely, that maybe some of a pharmacological agent's metabolites, that are not psychoactive, do have other somatic and biological adverse effects.

WB: Do you remember when you published your first paper, or presented it?

LG: Oh yes, I think that was, probably, out of medical school and that was in psychosomatic medicine and that was, probably, this was not in psychoactive drugs, but it was in Basal Motor Conditioning in Human Subjects. I did some of the research while I was a medical student. We found out that some people, using a classical condition, are very easily conditioned to have basal constriction and you measure their blood flow in their fingers with one or two shock treatments and some or not, just shocked, and that got published, I think, around 1946 or something of that sort. We're pretty proud of it and it probably does have some importance that we are quite different about our capacity to be conditioned and this was a condition response to turning on a light and some people, who were conditioned just to a couple of reinforcements, continued to have basic constriction if a light was turned on, I can imagine. No wonder some people get bad hypertension and some don't. There are probably genetic and other differences.

WB: Now, I know you're still active in doing some research. Can you tell us a little bit about what you're doing now?

LG: Yes, I'm still involved and I'm delighted with our own department that we have a brain imaging center and I know you are, too, and we did do a fair number of studies on brain imaging and PET scans and did look at the relationship of the anxiety and hostility and dreams, or when one is awake, to the PET scans and I, recently, with Ernest Noble, who was formerly at UCI, we've done a study with PET scan, showing that people with the A1 allele, who are normal, and who have no psychiatric history, their family or themselves, of drug abuse, or alcoholism, or obesity, have significantly different PET scans from people who don't have that allele. And, we would have never been able to do that, if we hadn't had a PET scan in our own backyard. That was one study. Another study that, in a way, I think is related to neuropsychopharmacology, it'll be interesting to see, but, rather by accident, published something in 1991, showing that, of all things, that manganese was elevated in the hair of violent criminals, as compared to controls. I didn't think much of that paper, but we published it, because there was no question about the finding. I didn't believe it the first time. I thought it was chance, for a sample, so we got another sample of criminals and controls and it showed up in the second sample. And, I was still pretty skeptical, being a Missouri boy, the Show Me state.

And, so, we got a third sample and it showed up again. The puzzling thing about the paper and the finding was, we had imperial findings without any hypothesis. And, since then, the Japanese and others have shown, well, the manganese does lower the serotonin level in the brain, rats, and there have a number of other studies, replicating our finding. And, we applied for a grant. This time, it's not usual, neuropsychopharmacological research but I guess that we're having it, in finding a place to send it, it's going to be the neurochemistry and biochemistry portion of NIMH. And, I can't believe that one little element would be a big factor in the problems that we're plagued with in our society with violence, but it may make some contribution. So, we're into that. There, the research is going to have to be, and I'm not unhappy about it, and it's going to have to be animal research, where we can control everything. That's one area. Another area that came back and it does relate to the content analysis, there was an advertisement by the National Institute on Drug Abuse, requesting a grant on computerized neuropsychiatric testing software. Well, I thought, that was just built for us. And, what they want is a software that will pick up a cognitive impairment in people that have been involved in drug abuse, so we've gone far. Whether we'll get it or not is something else. One way or the other we're going to do that. We're into that area and I think we have a pretty good chance to get the grant. Who knows?

WB: Well, I often think, once a researcher, always a researcher. It's impressive that you've, how many papers have you published?

LG: Well, I've got over two hundred papers and two hundred journal articles and about eighteen to twenty books.

WB: Well, it's impressive that a fifty year span and you're still going strong.

LG: I have a problem and I bet Bunney's are going to have it, namely, I wouldn't know how to retire. I think it's a problem.

WB: Yeah, okay. Now, who were some of the important people, not just in the beginning of your work, but along the way, that, I guess, you interacted with, working in the same area where colleagues were important for you to communicate with?

LG: Well, over the years. I'm still going to flash back to some of those mentors, back at Washington U and in Chicago, and they'd certainly get internalized; I was so probably carried away by then, that they're with me.

WB: You still see the influence of psychoanalysis though, you know. You have this concept of internalized, which I happen to believe in.

LG: Well, by internalized, I know I'm taking that word, but by internalized I mean that they're in my protein substance in my brain. In that sense, I didn't mean that.

WB: I know what you mean.

LG: And, the psychoanalysis thing, although, I'm still a training analyst, I must say that I figure that it's pretty much an art form, rather, and I'm disappointed that it didn't, it hasn't lent itself for most people to empirical approach. But, it probably has influenced my willingness to listen to people for a long time, as it probably has influenced you. By internalize, I mean in a biochemical way. Oh, I think of various people, they're, say in Cincinnati, Arthur Mersky, a biochemically oriented researcher, Maurice Levine, for that matter, although, he made it possible for me to do research and encouraging. But, at the University of California at Irvine, there were many people there in the medical school that made it possible to do research and to try to run a department. As a matter of fact, if I hadn't been able to do research, I don't think I would have been able to tolerate the administrative problems. There have been a lot of people involved in looking at the relationship of pharmacokinetics and chemical response and I edited two books on the topic and these were both under the imprimatur of the American College of Neuropsychopharmacology. It isn't a big or very important area these days. I can think of other people in that area, Alexander Glassman, but I wouldn't do him justice if I, to those authors that also were, whose chapters I'd published. I don't recall them right now. I'm impressed by this particular meeting, because I don't think it's that hot an area, although, it's an important thing and everybody does get blood levels, but what carries me away here is the genetics and its role in psychoactive drugs and so on.

WB: What would you consider, if you had to list one thing, what would you consider your biggest contribution to the field of science?

LG: It's hard to pick one thing, but if I had to think of it, it's a preoccupation with the accuracy and the precision of measurement, whether it's a measurement of psychological states and traits or from speech or the accuracy of measurement from blood levels of psychoactive drugs, you know, arranging from radioimmune assay to gas chromatographics. I think I've been occupied with developing or asking for the best and most precise ingenuous methods of measurement. It seems to me a lot of big discoveries have been made, you know. They've got the microscope or the telescope. You were instrumental in bringing a brain imaging center to UCI and I'm fascinated by that. I can't say that, that's my contribution, but I go that way. And, I do question the accuracy of the measurements, so I think a tremendous curiosity and insistence on objective and accurate measurements is one of my contributions.

WB: Okay. Were there any times that you were tempted to leave science, to leave research, job offers that would have taken you, either, out of the field or into too much administration?

LG: No, I, just like today, I mean, I can't imagine life, retirement and not doing science. And, administration, I had a taste of it. It was fun to have the opportunity to develop a department and get it started, but I've avoided positions of too much administration, because I thought it would take me away from science.

WB: Well, you were the founding Chair?

LG: Right.

WB: At the University of California, Irvine, Department of Psychiatry.

LG: And, I notice that you, too, are able to keep your activities into the science area and avoid too much administration. It takes one to know one.

WB: Are you pleased the way things have turned out or unhappy?

LG: Oh, you mean in my career?

WB: Your career.

LG: I'm pleased the way it's worked and the present and the way it's working. I have the phobia of retirement and I think I'll keep going as long as I can, because it's such a fascinating field. I can't think of anything more fascinating.

WB: Okay, now, where do you see that you've worked in or the field in neuropsychopharmacology, where do you see it going in the future. What's in the realistic future. What's in the blue sky future? What's your vision?

LG: Well, I think, in one area that I've made a very original contribution and that is the diagnosis of mental disorders and nervous problems. From language, I think, eventually, that's going to be possible from just voice recognition, using, they almost to have to use.....

WB: What do you mean by voice recognition?

LG: Well, here I'm talking here and the way that my content analysis measure works is, the material is tape recorded and, then, the type script put on a diskette and that's into word perfect and that's put into the computer and that comes up with all these scores in twelve different scales. There's one awkward step there.

WB: You mean, like anxiety and depression, that kind?

LG: Anxiety, how schizophrenic a bout is, how much cognitive environment and psychosis and the trouble is, that takes time. Somebody has to type what is said. I think it's going to be possible, in time, to take speech and, even with my hesitations here, because that gets scored, too, to directly program that for the computer so they can be analyzed.

WB: Without the typing, intermediate.

LG: Without the typing. Yeah. And, that's being done now. The problem is, the computer has to learn somebody's language. We're getting new software. Well, I got software a couple of years ago from IBM and it was very picky and finicky and had to do that. We're going to get new software. It's going to be broader, but the advances in computer technology are so fast that I think that's going to be relevant. You can think, well, what's that got to do with neuropsychopharmacology? Well, it's going to shorten some aspects of the diagnos is, but it's going to make it more precise and combining that with the very amazing and encouraging advances in translating genetic differences to understanding of the differences between these various organisms, it's going to help us predict what people are especially vulnerable. And, I do think there's going to be a combination of this more successful application of drugs and treatments for individuals and it's going to be a combination of these things. And, our technology is really going places. The biggest problem is going to be, can it be funded properly, but that's another question, but I'm a strong believer that we're on the right track. We're making tremendous advances, not just in psychiatric illnesses, but in programs like this. Some of the illnesses are neurological, say, multiple sclerosis and so on, and the interaction of genetic and environmental factors are well attended to. So, I'm very optimistic that we're going to continue to see tremendous advances in our field here.

WB: You see a more accurate diagnosis, a more accurate tailoring, then, a more accurate tailoring of active treatment potentials, modalities kind of exactly, in the future, and, then, eventually, an impact of genetics.

LG: Right.

WB: Now, what have I left out? What area are the things that I've left out?

LG: I think you've covered everything.

WB: That you want to put on the record?

LG: No, I think you've covered things very well. I really don't have much more to say, except I'm riding high on the continuing opportunity to do research and very happy that, at least in my genes, I guess, the Alzheimer's gene is absent or they're not playing a big part. I think it's very fortunate and I thank whoever is responsible for this.

WB: Okay. So, I've been interviewing, today, Dr. Louis Gottschalk, Professor at UCI. He has a distinguished career, spanning over fifty years from free neuroleptic drugs through to the present time. He continues, actively, in research. He's known many of the great people in the field of neuropsychopharmacology and it's been an honor to interview him.

LG: Thank you very much, Biff.

APRIL 1999

Interviewed by: Dr. Thomas Ban (TB).M.D., Professor Emeritus, Vanderbilt University, Nashville, Tennessee

TB: I am interviewing Dr. Louis Gottschalk for the American College of Neuropsychopharmacology (ACNP). He has been a member of the ACNP from the very beginning (1961). I am Thomas Ban and I think we are just going to start and go through with Dr. Gottschalk about his numerous contributions. With all this, I would like to add that we must look at Dr. Gottschalk as a psychiatrist, who during his academic and scientific career, covered all the different aspects of American psychiatry. He started with psychiatry and neurology and later with psychoanalysis and moved in all the different periods through American psychiatry and is active, even today. He is doing work with computerized content analysis of speech and verbal texts in order to achieve the measurement of neuropsychiatric states and traits. So we are going to see a very, very unique kind of life, which is, not only, reflecting a man but it reflects the whole period of American psychiatry, during the past fifty years. So, I think we can start and I really would to start at the very beginning, if you don't mind. Where were you born? What were your earliest kinds of experiences, what, you think, you know, you would like to share with us? We would like to hear, really, the different influences you had, your interests in your childhood and a little bit about your early education.

LG: I was born in St. Louis, Missouri, August 26, 1916. I was the third of four sons. My father was Max Wilhelm Gottschalk and my mother was Kelmie Mutrux Gottschalk. Father was born in the United States of German and Prussian background on his father's side and German and Austrian background on his mother's side.. My mother was of French-Swiss background, born in the United States. I mention those small details to indicate that I'm, maybe, a typical mixed ethnic background American, as many Americans are. I grew up in St. Louis and the parents, apparently, thought that, at best, the French-Swiss side, thought it was important for us children to learn to speak French and my maternal grandmother was still alive when I was born and we learned to speak in French, and it was spoken a great deal at home. And, some German, we heard occasionally. Father, I guess his parents spoke German, and he spoke German once in a while. I think it has some bearing on my life pattern, that my father was a very gifted man and like his own father, he was an obedient son and studied law and was a lawyer. His father was a lawyer, but as soon as my father, as I understand, finished getting his law degree, around the turn of the century, he didn't practice law. He had been taught to be a good musician and artist and, instead, he, as I understand, wrote for the St. Louis Post Dispatch, as an art and music critic, and he was a gifted musician, violinist, pianist and he tried composing for quartets, quintets and, even, opera, and he was a fine artist and was a good writer. I mention those things because the joy of just being creative had, with respect to my child rearing and development, certainly influenced us and was illustrated to us by my father. But, another side of the family, my mother's side of the family, Uncle Louis, who had twelve children, he, also, was in the same creative line and, as I understand, he saved his money and went to Paris to study art and came back to St. Louis and set up an art studio and couldn't make it, financially. But he did do pretty well in having children, conceived twelve of them. And, he became an architect and builder. I don't think one needed a license in those days. So, both sides of the family were artistic and musical. Creativity was encouraged.

I think, too, I wasn't very good at many of those things because I was third of four kids. They were all pretty good artists, so if we all sat around the table, we Gottschalk boys three years apart, or with my cousins, an older kid would often say, let's draw this or that. The stuff, I did, didn't seem very good compared to the older ones and the same with music; although, we all had to take music lessons. But there were, and I've reflected on this, casual, easy-going efforts to encourage us to write or be creative. And, I think that behavior got imprinted. One amusing story is that, when I was around four or five years of age, my father was talking with some friends of his in the kitchen, and they were talking about writing and so on, and I was copying what they were talking about, sitting there, scribbling on a piece of paper. I couldn't really write. And, one of my father's friends said, "This boy of yours, Louis, is writing". And, another one said, "What's he writing about"? And, he came over and said, "What are you writing about"? And, I said, "Writing a story". Well, he said, "Oh, fine. Read it to us". And, I read this scribble and they said, they didn't laugh or ridicule me, they said, "Very fine". So, I think, in a way, I was encouraged to write, even scribble, but encouraged, and, so, even if I do something in research and it doesn't pay off right away, well, I had fun doing it.

TB: Didn't you, actually, go into English at first; your first college study, wasn't it English?

LG: Well, I was growing up in the depression years (1928-1934) and my older brothers got to go to college, but by the time I came along, I couldn't. The family didn't have any money and I went to a public vocational school, learning secretarial skills and accounting. So, when I did finally go to College, I had a "Lust for Knowledge" there was a book by that name). I felt deprived and really eager to learn. I went to night school at Washington University and, a round-about way to answer your question, I didn't know what I wanted. I was just interested in everything that came along, whether it was English and Science. So, simultaneously, I was interested in English or the Sciences, not just English.

TB: Not just English?

LG: And, Foreign Language.

TB: So, your first degree that you had, what was it in?

LG: It was a Bachelor of Arts, but I took extra courses, I had a major in Biology and Psychology and English.

TB: I see, so, it was really a triple.

LG: Three—a triple major.

TB: Triple major, so it was even more than a double. Even then, you, really, you covered everything. Where did you, actually, go to college?

LG: I went to Washington University in St. Louis.

TB: St. Louis. It looks like, you see, that both your father and your mother's side, this had a big impact on all of you, right?

LG: Right.

TB: And, almost everything that happens, you know, in some way, parental influence are very strong.

LG: And, my father did have an interest in science. His brother, younger brother, Victor Hugo Gottschalk had a doctorate, a PhD, from the University of Chicago in Physics. So, the family was interested in the Arts and Sciences. It probably brushed off on me in some way.

TB: Obviously, it did. But, then, you immediately went from college, you continued in medical school. Am I correct?

LG: Yes, in medical school.

TB: And, very earlier, surely you got your College degree rapidly, right?

LG: No, I was delayed from high school and going to college, because of financial reasons, as I told you. Probably it wasn't all bad. There was about two and a half to three years lag before I went to college. I wasn't able to do so faster.

TB: I see.

LG: In that period of time, I brushed with the real world. I was a clerk in the First National Bank of St. Louis and I did a lot of other things. It probably was good for me. I was a little more mature, physically, and was really motivated then to go to college. I felt deprived and I was hungry for knowledge.

TB: And, you went to Washington.

LG: Washington University.

TB: And, apparently, during your medical school, Washington U. was an exceptionally good school, right? There are many excellent people that probably went there.

LG: Yes. I didn't realize how good it was, but I was certainly inspired in medical school. As an undergraduate at Washington U, I think I had some outstanding professors in English (Frank Webster, Dana Jensen), in Experimental Embryology (a Victor Hamburger). Professor Hamburger probably should have won a Nobel Prize. A Holly Compton, a Nobel Prize winner in Physics and, then, at Washington University Medical School, there were seven Nobel Prize winners. I just thought they were ordinary professors, but they were inspired and it brushed off on us.

TB: When in college, there were two Nobel Prizes, right? Who were they?

LG: One was Holly Compton.

TB: What did he actually do?

LG: He was a physicist. I can't say, exactly, why he got his prize. And, at medical school, there was Carl and Gerty Cori, biochemists, and there was a physiologist, James Erlanger. In any case, they were, not only fine researchers but very enthusiastic about what they did, and it brushed off on us.

TB: Oh, had you actually personal contact with any of them?

LG: Oh, yes, they were my professors.

TB: So, obviously. And, while you were at school with them, when did you decide to move into psychiatry or how did this happen?

LG: Well, the only reason I went to medical school, as a matter of fact, was to be a neuropsychiatrist.

TB: I see.

LG: I don't know how it happened, exactly, but I decided on that field before going to medical school. I was, you know, interested in the mind and the brain and why people behave the way they do. And I, even though there had been physicians in the family, I didn't know them. My main reason for going to medical school was to go into neuropsychiatry. And, I can't say exactly why.

TB: So, really, from the very beginning, you went to medical school because you wanted to deal with the brain and to do some research.

LG: Well, that was, also, to learn about human beings and why they think the way they do.

TB: And, it seems to be, you know, that you had a number of people who had a great impact on you. Is there anyone, especially, whom you would like to sort of, you know, bring to our attention, whom you had a very, very close contact during those years?

LG: Well, I should flash back just a moment, probably, to my undergraduate years. Well, there were some great professors there, Victor Hamburger (biology and experimental embryology), John Paul Nafe (physiological psychology), and a woman geneticist (whose name I can't recall at the moment.)., but my contemporaries, my classmates, I was surrounded by unusual people. I didn't realize it at the time. In addition, there was such people as Tennessee Williams, a classmate; William Inge, another playwright; Josephine Johnson, a Pulitzer Prize winner; Ed Meade, who wrote How to Succeed in Business Without Trying; and his younger brother. Walter Mead (another English major). And, I don't know why all those people, they were mostly English majors, happened to be there, but I was amongst them and I wrote for the college magazine (the Eliot) and college newspaper, and I think I enjoyed the fun of just writing or creating.

TB: You really had contact with Tennessee Williams?

LG: Yes, as an undergraduate. So, in medical school, I, also, then, didn't have the means to go but I got a break. By luck, I met the acting head of the department of Neuropsychiatry, a Dr. David Rioch, who was an extremely gifted neuroanatomist and neurologist and who wrote the section in Gray's Anatomy on the extrapyramidal system. And, he got me a job at Washington U. in the Department of Neuropsychiatry; it was a combination of neurology and psychiatry, and a Josiah Macy Foundation Fellowship that paid seventy-five dollars a month. Well, that made it possible to go to medical school and I, probably, was one of the only few people in the class that had an outside job. But I worked there in the Neuropsychiatry department, and I can visualize very clearly all those people. There was David Rioch, doing research. I was assigned to a Dr. Felix Deutsch, M.D., a famous doctor. Anna Deutsch, his wife was a famous psychoanalyst and wrote on the psychology of women. He was a psychoanalyst and had been a physiatrist, physical medicine. There was John Whitehorn, who became the Chair of the department, was a psychiatrist who had done biochemistry and developed a test for chlorides. There was another person like him from Yale University, who later became the Chairman, Dr. Edwin Gildea, who had a degree in biochemistry, as well as psychiatry; a George Bishop, physiologist, who set a rare example. How did he get famous? He was interested in nerves and skin and he tested in his own hand and his arms, all the points that would make you feel temperature or touch or pain and, then, on his own hand he dissected each different area. And he was credited with discovering and describing the peculiar little receptors and organs for those sensations from the skin. And, I thought, my goodness, man, he uses a piece of himself to discover this. And, there were other examples around there. I had a couple of assistant professors that had come from Harvard, a George

Saslow, who later became Chairman of Psychiatry at Oregon State University and Daniel Badal, who later became a Professor at the University of Cleveland. And those young men, (It doesn't seem to happen today, anymore), competed with one another for the opportunity and time in their efforts to teach us. We had just a few psychiatric residents, that time.

TB: It was very stimulating.

LG: Very stimulating!

TB: Very stimulating, but it seems to me you went immediately after medical school, when you got your degree, immediately to psychiatry residency, am I correct?

LG: Yes, well, I hadn't realized it, but because I was an honor student and Phi Beta Kappa and Alpha Omega Alpha, I was offered an internship in surgery or medicine. I took the internship in straight medicine. It was competitive. There was a Chairman of Medicine in the medical school, Dr. Barry Wood, a very good Professor, who later became famous. And, I think you still have to do so, you had to have a year of internship. I took straight medicine internship and after I took that, I was offered a residency to stay in medicine. But I was still hooked on neuropsychiatry. And, I turned it down, same as I did surgery. Those were supposed to be great honors, but I was interested in that strange field of neuropsychiatry.

TB: So, you had a straight medical internship. You reverted to psychiatry. Am I correct, you were the Chief Resident of Neuropsychiatry?

LG: I became the Chief Resident.

TB: And after you completed your neuropsychiatric training you started psychoanalysis, training in psychoanalysis.

LG: I didn't start in psychoanalysis. I really started in psychiatry and neurology, and it was later that I got into psychoanalysis. Those were the war years, World War II. I graduated. I went to medical school from 1940 to 1943, December, and they speeded up the time required for medical school and residency training. We had no summer vacations and the last year of medical school, we were drafted into the military, but deferred so that we could finish our medical school and, then, be of military service. I selected what I wanted to do and I had that internship in medicine and neuropsychiatry residency. And, as soon as they could they put us to work in our medical specialty, neuropsychiatry. They were lots of neuropsychiatric casualties and, so, we went, immediately, after residency, into military service. That was 1946, and I was in the United States Public Health Service and I went to the United States Public Health Service Hospital in Fort Worth, Texas, a two thousand bed hospital on ten thousand acres. It had been a narcotic hospital,for the Public Health Service, but it was turned over to, (it's a huge place), the Navy and Marine Corp, Coast Guard and Merchant Seaman for neuropsychiatric casualties that they didn't have room for elsewhere. And, so, I was there for two years. There were a number of U.S. Public Health Service docs, who had become militarized. It's usually a peace time service, working in collaboration with doctors from the Navy and Marine Corps. And we each had these huge patient loads of about a hundred and twenty patients, about thirty new patients a month. So, I was there for about two years and, then, it was after that, because I was a hard-working public health service officer. Around that time, the federal government and, I guess, the United States Public Health Service, was planning the Institutes of Medicine and the National Institute of Mental Health. And, it so happened, there were, I guess, officers there in Texas and Washington, D.C. that said, "Well, this might be a good man to recruit to be a psychiatrist at the National Institute of Mental Health". And, I suppose, the buildings weren't ready in Washington, D.C., so, they said, "Well, you can have another two or three years of training, whatever you want, anywhere you want to go." And, at that time, I had in my mind to, probably, because of the example of one of my younger mentors (Dr. Daniel Badal), who had neurosurgical training before he switched over to neuropsychiatry at Harvard. I thought, well, my goodness, I'll get a neurosurgical residency. And, at the same time, because of one of my older mentors, Ed Gildea, said, "Well, if you are interested in psychotherapy, it wouldn't be a bad idea to get some psychoanalytic training. At least, they listen to people a long time". He was conservative about it and, so, that's why I happened to got to Chicago and applied for a neurosurgical residency at the Illinois Neuropsychiatric Institute and to the Chairman of Neurosurgery there. He said to me: "you're already trained in neurology and psychiatry. I don't know why you want psychoanalytic training, but as far as getting neurosurgical training, I don't know whether those are compatible, neurosurgery and psychoanalysis". And, he turned me down. I said to him: "Well, it won't cost you any money, because the United States Public Health Service is going to pay for all this training." That didn't persuade him. (He didn't know what a good man he was losing, but maybe it was lucky for me.) Well, I went to see Roy Grinker, a famous neurologist and psychiatrist, and he offered me training in child psychiatry. That's how I got into child psychiatry. And, I did psychoanalytic training, then, beginning around 1948, in child psychiatry, adult and child analysis, at the Chicago Psychoanalytic Institute. In that setting, being interested in the brain and the mind at the same time, those were not incompatible areas. Grinker was a famous neurologist who had had a psychoanalysis with Sigmund Freud. And there was at the University of Illinois and University of Chicago, they gave doctorate education in Neurophysiology and for some reason or other, at that time, any compatibility between psychoanalysis and neurophysiology didn't exist. Some people got both. So, I was exposed to that.

TB: The chronology, you graduated from medical school in '43, am I correct?

LG: Yes, graduated from medical school in '43.

TB: Then, you went to the United States Public Health Service which was militarized and after a couple of years at the USPHS hospital in Fort Worth, Texas where you diagnosed and treated neuropsychiatric casualties from World War II, you were offered a position at the National Institute of Mental Health. You were going to be ready to perform as a psychiatrist, research psychiatrist. And you were recruited way in advance and even before you had your training in child psychiatry and psychoanalysis.

LG: Yes.

TB: And, then, instead of becoming a neurosurgeon, because there was too much doubt in the mind of a director of neurosurgery about the compatibility of neurosurgery and psychoanalysis, you went into child psychiatry and, at the same time, analytic training. But, by that time, am I correct, you already had some involvement in psychophysiology and electroencephalography? You had already published your first paper, when was that and how did it happen?

LG: It was published in 1946, in Psychosomatic Medicine and that was on producing conditioned vasomotor responses in ten human subjects using photoelectric plethysmography and that was done at Washington U. It was probably my combining some of the teachings of a couple of my professors. One was Carlyle Jacobson, who was another professor there, a physiological psychologist, who got me to reading all I could about conditioning and behavior and Pavlovian conditioning. And that's how I got into that project, but it was, also, carried out under the influence of somebody that I'd see at the other end of the scale of continuity, and that was Felix Deutsch. I was being a research assistant in some research he was doing. He had a photoelectric plethysmograph, a device that would pick up the blood flow in the finger, and I got the idea, on my own. I thought of producing conditioned vasomotor responses in people and see whether their peripheral vascular system could be conditioned, and see if I could produce a vasoconstriction within the fingers in response to a faradic stimulus, on the other hand, and see whether there is any difference in people who condition rapidly, and those who don't.

TB: So, what were the conditional and what were the unconditional actually?

LG: Well, as I say, a faradic stimulus in a light.

TB: In a light.

LG: Light on the ceiling.

TB: So, you really conditioned vasomotor constriction to the light?

LG: Right. I found that some people, I figure it's still a non-important piece of work, they show that, somehow, among ten individuals, some condition very rapidly, after one or two reinforcements and, then, they show extinction of the condition response and some subjects were very hard to condition. And I think it probably shows that some of us have a genetic propensity, to have conditioned vascular responses.

TB: So, you really had acquisition and extinction. Did you have any other conditional features in this research?

LG: There was a questionnaire. I had a questionnaire in order to study, somewhat, the vascular feelings and the emotional feelings of these people. And the subjects, as I remember, who had more variability in awareness of emotional differences were more easily conditioned. I did figure, you know, some of us have a higher vulnerability to vascular disturbances than others.

TB: What was really the hypotheses? You were using this plethysmographic method with a vasomotor conditioning, but when you set up your project, what was the hypothesis?

LG: Well, the hypotheses were: can vasomotor conditioning be achieved in human subjects and are there any differences in individuals who condition rapidly and those who don't? And, when I was reading Pavlov, some dogs got easily conditioned to salivary response and some didn't. And, I wondered, is that how it happens in humans?

TB: But, you really didn't try to link it to the temperament of types.

LG: No.

TB: You really didn't; you could have done anything.

LG: True. I had a two-tailed test; let's see whether there is any difference and is there any? I knew there were differences in temperament.

TB: But, actually, to both. At any rate, you had a questionnaire and you tried to link the vasomotor conditioning you found to emotional variables; so you tried to link it to visuo-motor characteristics.

LG: And, that could be said to be temperament, in a way.

TB: Yes, whatever. But, that's pretty much what this was, am I correct? Your first publication and you did it, completely, yourself. I suppose you set up your instruments and everything.

LG: Yes. I had to do all this while I was working as a house officer and attending medical school. You know, I had med school and house officer responsibilities. And, I was in a, say, in a cordial environment. The department of psychiatry fostered my doing that.

TB: Who was the Chairman?

LG: Well, as I said, at first, it was John Whitehorn and later on, he became department Chairman at Hopkins. And he was followed by Edwin Gildea.

TB: So, these were the two Chairmans, in fact, during that period.

LG: During that period, yes.

TB: And, after this residency, where did you do your child psychiatry?

LG: Well, at Michael Reese in Chicago.

TB: Michael Reese.

LG: Right.

TB: And, parallel with that, you did your psychoanalysis.

LG: Exactly.

TB: And, immediately, when you had both, you went to NIMH, you joined NIMH. At the first, actually, as a research psychiatrist.

LG: First research psychiatrist in 1951.

TB: Who did you work with? You were at NIMH. Whom did you recruit?

LG: I wasn't into recruiting, that was not my job, but I can say who was there.

TB: Who was there?.

LG: Who was running the institute, actually, was a doctor who had been, for a short time, at the United States Public Health Hospital in Texas, a Dr. Robert Felix.

TB: Robert Felix, he was the first director, right?

LG: First director and I was the first research psychiatrist there. There was a neurophysiologist there, Wade Marshall, Ph.D., who learned that when I was in Chicago, I had done studies with epileptic children, and he thought maybe he could collaborate with me. He said, while he was doing studies, placing aluminum gel on the brains of animals to make them more susceptible to having epileptic seizures, since they already had seizures. He said you had to chase them around and beat them a little bit in order to have them have seizures. He wondered whether maybe that's the part that I might want to do, irritating the animals. So they have seizures. And, I said, "No, thanks". I was free to do whatever research I might want to do.

TB: Whatever you wanted to do.

LG: Yes. Take out and do whatever I wanted to do. It still works that way, I think.

TB: But, you had to be very much involved by then, if I am correct is the question? I have a feeling that you were also involved very early in EEG, in electroencephalography. In fact, am I correct that you made some contribution to the nasal pharyngeal kind of lead?

LG: While I was at the United States Public Health Service Hospital, a couple of years there, they had this huge hospital, they wanted somebody to run the EEG machine and laboratory there in the department. And they let me go back to Washington U. for a couple of months to learn more about electroencephalography. And, I already knew some, but, I mean, I focused on it a couple of months with James O'Leary and George Bishop. I suppose that was a relatively new procedure back in those days. It wasn't absolutely new. But, in any case, when I was at the Public Health Service Hospital, for the last six months, I looked over and reviewed their EEG's. And, then, when I transferred to Michael Reese Hospital, I got involved with their their EEG's; I got into reviewing them. And, it was there, though, having studied these children, I got into asking the Clinical Services for children at Michael Reese, who had epilepsy, who were being treated in the epilepsy clinic, and I asked to see some of the children, in which the anticonvulsant medication didn't control their seizures. I saw a number of them and decided to treat them, a selected few of them with psychotherapy and/or play therapy.

But also, one of my first control cases in child analysis, I had accepted a five-year-old Polish Catholic boy, who had seizures not inhibited by anticonvulsant medication of any kind, and I got the idea to see whether child analysis had any favorable effect. We were really sold those days on the power of psychoanalysis and child analysis. On that case, that's how I happened to get into research into the psychological trigger mechanisms of epilepsy. I think I wrote that up somewhere. That little boy did get better; his seizures stopped. I saw him about four times a week and, you know, very classical psychoanalysis. And, there's another I child I saw, an eight-year-old boy, and he would look through a window screen and could bring on a seizure. And, I wrote his case up and that was published in the Psychoanalytic Study of the Child. Well, from that experience, I won the Hofheimer Prize for Research in Psychiatry. I got the idea of looking for the trigger process of the seizures in those kids. In this little Polish boy, in his play therapy and seeing his problems about making noise and so on, he got over his seizures, and I followed that case for many years.

TB: You mentioned the Hofheimer Prize, actually, for this epileptic type work. When did this happen? When did you?

LG: Well, this was back, about, probably, 1955.

TB: Well, this was a little bit later where we, actually, are. This is perfectly fine. So, really, after this training in psychoanalysis and child psychiatry, you moved to NIMH.

LG: NIMH.

TB: And, you worked, mainly, with epilepsy, am I correct?

LG: Yes. I decided, well, what I am I going to do up here? Well, it so happened, when I try to continue what I'm working on and, it so happened, that Dr. David Rioch, who had been one of my mentors and guides at Washington U., was, now, head of neuropsychiatry at Walter Reed Army Hospital. And, I thought, well, suppose I look him up and tell him what my idea is and what I want to do. I did so, and, he made it possible. He said, "Well, you can study inpatients here. We have some military inpatients that have seizures and you can use these patients. Why don't you study them?" So, that's how I happened to get into and, then, setting up things there, I had the idea, well, let's pick individuals with these seizures; I saw a lot of them; who have recurring abnormal EEG paroxysms and EEG waves, who may not have seizures or visible seizures, and, then I interviewed them. This was an attempt to combine free associations with neurophysiological findings and I did that for awhile. I did find the right kind of patients. I still have records on them. And, I got the feeling of, that it was very easy to identify these abnormal EEG paroxysms. It's very clear cut. But the other side of the research, that is, listening and taking the recordings of what they say, there isn't very much objective science in that process.

TB: Am I correct that you were trying to combine three things, in a way, or even four, because it was your training in psychoanalysis, as well, which included free association, to use whatever you can use through the free association? You had your great interest in techniques like electroencephalography and these types of things.

LG: And a nasal pharyngeal electrode for EEG recording.

TB: A nasal pharyngeal electrode, because you really moved into electroencephalography, am I correct, you were the first one, am I correct, to fashion one? So, you really moved and sort of invented something.

LG: Never give up.

TB: Yes, try something. And, then, you even combined your conditioning experience, your background in vasomotor conditioning research and experience to study the psychopathogenesis of epileptic seizures, right? So, all of this, you tried to combine and tried to see what can one learn from, am I correct?

LG: Exactly, Tom.

TB: Now, we are, treatment-wise, in epilepsy, because one of your research areas has been epilepsy because you feel that seizures involve the neurologist, am I correct?

LG: You are correct.

TB: Now, what was, actually, the pharmacological treatment during those days of epilepsy?

LG: There are a variety anticonvulsant medications, including dilantin and the barbiturates.

TB: We are probably in that period, early fifties, right, we were moving toward the mid fifties. You are still at NIMH. At the same time, you are collaborating with your former Chairman's department of Neuropsychiatry at Washington University, right?

LG: Well, David Rioch was Chairman, but he made it possible for me to see patients at Walter Reed.

TB: Yes. How long did you stay at NIMH?

LG: Only a couple of years.

TB: Couple of years, so this means '51 to '53, right?

LG: Exactly right.

TB: Where did you go from NIMH?

LG: I was married. I had two children and I was married to a very gifted and beautiful doctor, Helen Reller, and she was a dermatologist and we were very happy. And we decided we wanted more children. We had two. I wanted a larger family and the United States Public Health Service, even though, we were both well trained and we had American Boards in our medical specialties, I had a relatively small income, and I asked my USPHS superiors whether it was possible for me to do any private medical practice to supplement my USPHS salary. They wouldn't let me and, so, I decided, well, the environment is great but my income is too small, I was offered, I didn't seek it, but I was offered a position at the University of Cincinnati. I had no idea of going there but, at that time, the University of Cincinnati and Cincinnati General Hospital was one of the top places to go for psychosomatic research. They had some famous people there.

TB: Who was the Chairman?

LG: Maurice Levine.

TB: Maurice Levine, right.

LG: There were other people of scientific note there, Arthur Mirsky for one.

TB: Paul Ornstein?

LG: Well, he was just a psychiatric resident when I first went there. He was not that famous and he was just a resident. How do you know Paul Ornstein? He was one of my analysands, in psychoanalytic training.

TB: He was Hungarian. But, you know, Heinz Lehman used to go there and I wrote in psychopharmacology.

LG: I'll tell you who else was there, George Engel and Arthur Mirsky. That could be a congenial place for psychosomatic research, because I was into that. Paul Ornstein didn't come along till much later and, as a matter of fact, he was interested in psychoanalysis and I turned out later to be his training analyst.

TB: I didn't know that.

LG: I was his training analyst. I knew his poor wife, Anna Ornstein, who was in a Nazi prison camp.

TB: Actually, in psychopharmacology at that time, it was Dr. Douglas Goldman in Cincinnati.

LG: Yes, right.

TB: Yes, there was Goldman.

LG: I knew him very well, sure. But he wasn't in the Department of Psychiatry at the University of Cincinnati..

TB: Because, you know, he was really already very much involved in using drug treatment. Did you have any contact?

LG: Oh, yes. I knew him very well. He was right in the forefront of drugs, but using them a great deal, but not in a discriminating way. You know, he didn't use these placebo-drug control studies. He just was an enthusiast. But he was not on the faculty.

TB: But, he was very much involved.

LG: He didn't do any hard experimental work. It was clinical treatment.

TB: Yes, he was a clinician. So, in fact, I have a feeling that toward the end, he really primarily had a very large practice.

LG: Oh, yes, he always had a big practice.

TB: He was just very much in the forefront with chlorpromazine and with any of the new drugs in that period. And, this was not as popular.

LG: Well, in some cities, it was. But, he was quite active.

TB: Quite active in it. So, any way, were there other researchers there?

LG: You probably don't know Arthur Mirsky.

TB: I did.

LG: Oh, you did. He was the biochemist who was interested in psychoanalysis and made some interesting contributions.

TB: Would you like to elaborate a little bit on him, or did you work with him, together?

LG: I didn't do any collaborative research.

TB: You didn't do any.

LG: No, but I was certainly a friend of his and he went to Chicago Institute for Psychoanalysis.

TB: Well, actually, there are many kinds of aspects of work where there are some collaboration, because, you know, you were trying to use psychoanalysis, not necessarily biochemistry. You were trying more to use with imaging and with neurophysiology.

LG: Yes. Well, that's one of the reasons I let myself go to Cincinnati, because there was some congenial research people on the facuty. George Engel was another internist that got interested in psychoanalysis. He was an identical twin and he got into psychoanalysis. He outlived his identical twin.

TB: Well, what was, really, your position in Cincinnati?

LG: I was, at first, research associate professor and later, research professor.

TB: And, this is where, actually, you went to the University of California at Irvine. So, you really did not move as much as some people do. You went straight from NIMH to Cincinnati.

LG: Wait a minute. I started in St. Louis, went to Fort Worth, Texas; then I went to Chicago.

TB: What did you do in Fort Worth?

LG: I told you, that's where I said I had to go from St. Louis to the military service. So I had to go to Fort Worth, Texas and from Fort Worth, Texas, I went to Chicago and from Chicago, I went to Bethesda, Maryland and, then, I moved to Cincinnati. It all depends on how you look at it, probably not moving as much as you, but you moved between two countries.

TB: I've moved much less, because all I moved was from Budapest to Montreal.

LG: But, I thought you went to Austria for a while.

TB: Oh, I had to wait for my boat to get across the Atlantic. I was just waiting.

LG: Oh, I thought you were in Vienna.

TB: I was in Vienna. You are very correct. I did the EEG's, some easy work at Allegemeines Krankenhaus, but, really you know, when you leave a country, it takes a little while until you get all your passports and they ship you. I was just waiting there.

LG: So, I, actually, moved, it seems very much to me, but over long periods of time.

TB: What I really meant to kind of say that, professionally, as soon as you completed your training, which I almost take it as your first real job in psychiatry was at NIMH, because everything was preparation. You did a little work before with Public Health, even publications, but after, then, Cincinnati and Irvine, right?

LG: You can put it that way. I look, however, at each place, as well as being in the federal government, as a job. When I became an intern and resident at Washington U, so, you know, I considered it was a real job. At Washington U, in those days, it was quite an honor to be made a medical house officer and I got ten dollars a month and white uniforms and food. And the second year I got twenty-five, and the third year I got seventy-five, almost enough to consider getting married. So, when you say, your first real job, hey, I got a salary at the United States of Public Health Service as a lieutenant commander and, then, I made big money. So, I'm looking at it that way.

TB: Yes, you were really high up.

LG: Well, the money was and it was, I'm sure you're aware of this, to go into the military, at that time in that war, all of us, who had been deferred, but most of us in the United States were committed to that war. We were willing to work as hard as we could to do something solid, as a real job.

TB: Well, it was, actually.

LG: And, then, the period in Chicago, I was on a military salary.

It was pretty good. And, on top of it, the extra good aspect of it was that you could do and get any other training you wanted to. You know, I think I mentioned yesterday, the United States Public Health Service, I think those top people were inducing other people to come aboard and if they wanted psychoanalysis that would be paid for. They'd pay for it. So, you know, an organically oriented person as Seymour Kety got psychoanalysis when he went to the NIMH. I don't know what he did with it, but you know, it was some experience he could get with his job.

TB: When did you get to, what year was it, actually, to Cincinnati, '54?

LG: 1953.

TB: 1953. So, it was '53, and you, really by that time, you had all kinds of papers, because was that anything which you think that you should mention. What you think, we already mentioned, basically, we mentioned the vasomotor conditioning.

LG: It was at the National Institute of Mental Health, while I was there, where I had the luxury of doing anything in research that I wanted to study. You know, it was a researcher's dream. I decided that what needed more study, and I might be a good person to do that, was to try to objectify the diagnosing of mental state or psychological or psychobiological feelings from language. Having looked at that and trying to put together those free-associations, what people were saying, and their abnormal EEG paroxysms burst from their brain waves, I got the idea of pursuing language and seeing whether I could objectify that more. I started out with, actually, taking movies of people and, actually, with a younger colleague of mine, Dr. Gove Hambidge. We did a couple of papers together. We tried to put everything together, movement, tone of voice and what they said, the semantics, and I realized this was beyond a promising schedule. But our work was published.

TB: But, did I understand correctly, Gove Hambidge, who did you mention?

LG: Gove Hambidge, who had also been at the United States Public Health Service hospital in Fort Worth, Texas, and who, they, also, gave this opportunity to go to NIMH. He had been a graduate of Yale Medical School, and, then, they let him have a psychoanalysis in New York City. And, so, after I was at NIMH, he joined me about six months later. I stuck to working on the content analysis of verbal behavior. He didn't. You know, he left and never did go back to it.

TB: So, really, your Content Analysis started over at the NIMH, right?

LG: Right.

TB: Now, then, you moved to Cincinnati and this time, I suppose, steadily continued.

LG: Yes, having been at NIMH and knowing something the problems and the challenges of applying for research money, even, when you're in an intramural research situation, is not easy. But, I was programmed and I applied for various research grants and got some. Among those was a grant, which I got, an RO research project on content analysis of language. And I tried other ones, which I got. And, then, I also later, in about five or six years, tried, because I was getting some prominence in research, I tried for a Research Career Award and I got a Research Career Award. It gave me, I wouldn't say a lot of money, but it gave me time to try to make a living for four kids and, also, try to do some research.

TB: So, you really got into this language in the early fifties, '52, '53, right? How did you get to language, because this had to be a crucial, this was probably one of the most crucial kind of decisions?

LG: As I say, I like to write. I like to listen to language and you're a psychiatrist, yourself, how do psychiatrists learn anything about anybody? They do what you're doing right now, asking questions and listening and trying to make something of the language. I had some interest in language, anyway, to some extent, foreign languages. I spoke a bit of French. In those days, an American med student had to have German. I studied German and, so, languages interested met, but I thought it was easy just to, on the surface of it, to say, well, how do all these skillful people arrive at conclusions about how somebody else feels. Now, in Chicago, they often argued about that. There was one other mentor, Franz Alexander, and a fellow countryman of yours and other people that argued out out lond what a person was communicating. They'd argue about what a patient was saying to me. I figured, well, here's a great scientist, but it's black and white; why do they have to argue? Well, I, later, found out, they just liked to argue, even, when they agreed. But, in any case, I think that got me into it and it wasn't an obsession. I stuck to it. It was, when you're trying to make an assessment of somebody's feelings, or a diagnosis, you can either use a psychiatric interview; you can use an adjective checklist; you can use a Beck Depression Inventory, or is there any other way to do it? Is there something scientific, since people differ a lot about how they check these adjective checklists. I mean, the reliability, sometimes, is pretty poor. And, so, that just pushed me on to see whether I could improve on this measurement problem. I had no idea, when I was working on it, it would go as far as it did. I think the wise choice I made, going back about twenty-five years ago, after we did prove that we could do Content Analysis of Language and made headway in reliability and validity, was to try to computerize the measurement methodology. And, that was a lucky thing, or maybe not lucky, but I thought, it takes so damn much time to try to figure out how to score these scales, according to the Gottschalk-Gleser Method, it's just like you have to go back to school. If it can be done by human, it should be possible to do it by machine, if there's really anything to it. And, I stuck to that. The first grant I applied for, back in 1975, and sent to NIMH, they sent it back. The pink sheet said, this can't be done, this can't be done. It's impossible to do this by machine.

TB: But, you see, this was, as I see it, from the off side, very much of your characteristic, because you were interested in quantification. You were, again, one of the first to pick up, that, basically, you should be able to use those computers in a meaningful kind of manner and tried, actually, to put it in, as much as possible.

LG: And, the same of mind, probably, was involved when I got into the drug blood levels in pharmacokinetics, just get numbers.

TB: Yeah.

LG: You know, it's not language, now, but it's the whole body and let's learn about pharmacokinetics and blood levels and what's all these things? It's something that's characterized my interest, you know, like brain waves, even, they had a problem, but how about Positron Emission Tomography, then, you end up in numbers?

TB: Which is, also, very consistent, actually, am I correct, you mathematize?

LG: Mathematize.

TB: Mathematize, that's right. But, you've had, somehow, you had that ability, you know, and you seek an interest and you pick up, you, really, just picked up everything, almost before it was really clearly expressed. You know, you had already picked it up, because, even, also, I think, if I'm correct, pharmacokinetics had been set up a bit later, around '60, '61, am I correct?

LG: Sure.

TB: Which is still one of, you know, very early. And, up to this point, you did your first psychopharmacology work, at this paper, which I know of in the mid sixties. Do you know which I am referring to, or which was, actually, your first paper, dealing with drugs?

LG: I have to check my CV, but I did, I think, in the fifties, probably, some studies.

TB: Your very first, if I am correct, you see, your first paper was Exploration of Testing Drugs Effecting Physical and Mental Activity.

LG: JAMA.

TB: Yes, this was in '56.

LG: '56.

TB: I really want to know what it was.

LG: It was pipradrol.

TB: It was pipradrol.

LG: You know that?

TB: Oh, yes.

LG: And, what I tried was, I got a group of pharmacologists and psychoanalysts, if people take a small dose of a medication like that, what's their reaction vs. a placebo? And, the interesting finding was that, well, how they experience it depends a lot on their personality. If somebody, I know they did and JAMA accepted it, if somebody is uncomfortable about being pushed to do something, instead of getting a pleasant feeling, they get anxious, depend by a drug, and if somebody is a little depressed or, you know, slow, we were talking about ADD, and they've liked to feel a little pushed inside, they feel better. And, the study showed, well, I mean in this a mixture of pharmacologists and psychoanalysts, psychiatry and psychiatric, the range of reactions to small doses was pretty large and it depended somewhat upon their general personality. You know, there are some people, as you well know, who have paradoxical reactions to drugs. So, that was the first paper.

TB: So, really, your first involvement in psychopharmacology was with pipradrol, really, am I correct? At least, in your biography?

LG: Probably, except, indirectly. I'm flashing back. Taking those kids in Chicago, who had seizures and they were on psychoactive drugs and anticonvulsant and the anticonvulsant worked some, but not perfectly. And, there the motivation was, well, either they had some incorrigible seizure or there's something else that's triggering the seizures and at a break, they break through. You know, like, we talked about, A. A. Wilson's articles about, some people, if they get angry, might get, also, real genuine seizures, no fake. So, indirectly, they're always saying, well, what's it again, the interaction of drugs and relief of symptoms.

TB: And, actually, you, also, did some pharmacological experiments, pharmacological with EEG, you know, like an early stage, if I am correct. But in a kind of systematic way, I think, the pipradrol, at least. Was it a placebo controlled study? It seems to be, it was placebo controlled.

LG: Yes. Not everybody had ever heard of pipradrol.

TB: No, but, you see at that time, it was quite popular and, you know, the story of metrazol and pentathol. And you have to had some exposure, also, to Ladislas Meduna, the originator of convulsive therapy for dementia praecox (schizophrenia). Did you know him?

LG: No, I didn't know him.

TB: You didn't know him?

LG: You didn't, did you?

TB: No, no.

LG: I just knew of him.

TB: I worked in the same place. I started psychiatry in the place where he introduced the use of metrazol to produce convulsions in mental patients.

LG: Really?

TB: Before.

LG: That was in Budapest?

TB: That was in Budapest.

LG: A few years before?

TB: A few years before, yes. I was a child when this happened. But, anyway, you are one of the few who worked with pipradrol and you worked with normal subjects. You did not work with them in geriatrics or any other population. And, you were really trying to connect it with personality dimensions. And since you didn't come from Hungary, because there is some kind of similar kind of research there. I don't recall now that I did research with pipradrol but I did it with stimulants and sedatives, vision and other dimensions.

LG: Personality and drug interactions.

TB: Interactions, right.

LG: Well, if you give a person a big enough, you might overwhelm the personality. But, I already had experience. Well I had some experience with colleagues, one good friend of mine. I won't mention his name, a psychiatrist. He asked me to be present when he had surgery for a gallbladder operation, because he was afraid of passivity. And, then, the anesthesiologists decided, well, they would give him a spinal. They were going to have to increase it. Well, it's just true, when they gave him a sedative, he got excited, paradoxically, instead of getting sedated. Yes, and it does happen, for example, the transient excitement just before going to sleep occurring with some slow-acting soporific drugs. It's demonstrable.

TB: What was your personality dimension, what you were using, actually, because you, obviously, used personality, some kind of personality dimensions with pipradrol?

LG: Which study is that?

TB: With the very first one. With pipradrol?

LG: No special test. I simply asked the subjects what their emotional reaction was, their reasoning and their emotional reactions.

TB: So, there was no special testing procedure.

LG: The questions I asked the subjects are documented precisely in the article.

TB: Oh, no, this is fine.

LG: Well, I was developing it, the content analysis methodology.

TB: Yes, at that point, you had already published your first major papers on the subject.

LG: I tried two approaches on the Content Analysis. One was, not entirely original, I don't think. I was just looking at words and not the meanings being communicated in a whole grammatical clause. I was looking at how many representative adjectives or verbs and so on, and I published some rather interesting papers using that approach. One on suicide notes and I demonstrated that you could distinguish real suicide notes (written by pen), from false suicide notes. That was in a study, I think it was promoted and organized by two suicide researchers on the topic of Are There Any Difference in False and Genuine Suicide Notes, and our work was published in Medical Psychology. There was a difference, but at the level of words. But, with that approach, I wondered whether I should stick it out there or should I look at the grammatical clause, the smallest unit of verbal communication. As I said, I later decided to focus on the grammatical clause because with regards to semantic units that most of us understand, the smallest unit is a grammatical clause. Sure, somebody could say, "damn" and it usually means "damn you", But taking words out of context can be unreliable for objective and valid findings. There was a group at Harvard that used just words, and they stuck to that approach. I mean, discounting the words depends how they're placed in a sentence. You know, there's a "damn you" or "damn myself" or "I hate". And, so, common sense will tell you, but in that whole field, Harvard got involved in using, there was a group there that got involved in using words and computers. The only thing is, it doesn't tell who's angry with whom and, so, I got into this other approach, sticking to the grammatical clause.

TB: Since this speech and content analysis will come back and back, will it be possible that just in two or three minutes, in a few sentences to arrive at a reliable and valid assessment?, If you could put it together, it would be an extraordinary achievement. I'm a creator now, just in a very simple way, because any people, in ten or twenty years or ten or fifty years, would find an achievement like that valuable.

LG: Well, Tom, I'll give it a shot. This is often the problem since I've been publishing in this area for, you know, twenty or twenty-five years, and that is, how to make this thing simple and understandable. Now, it turns out the whole process has grown, so it's got more and more complicated and, then, when I try to explain the procedure and how you can teach a dumb computer to do this, it is rather difficult. But, let me give it a shot. Because actually, if somebody with my type of mind or your type of mind is really interested in the details, well, in just looking at a TV like this, you're going to go to the original writings. That's what I do, to see what was said. But, in any case, because I have details of the methodology in a document right here, writing a research grant from the National Institutes of Health, and Research Review Committee, I'd better be sure and make it clear to them. But let me give it a shot. How can one, say, measure the magnitude of anxiety or the severity of schizophrenia or cognitive impairment from five minute speech samples? Well, one problem is, how can you standardize what somebody says? If I ask you, well, tell me about the good times you had and tell me about the bad times, you're going to give me some different language. So, the first step was to try to get a standard sample and to do so we borrowed some ideas from psychology—-namely, projection, specifically, the Thematic Apperception test. When one tries to give an individual a standard way to try to elicit the speech and, if one succeeds in doing so, one can use and compare verbal samples from other subjects and within a subject. On the other hand, one can use a verbal text somebody wants to study. Like the New York Times which changes its headlines daily over the past thirty years. You can compare the verbal content of those headlines, but if you're going to try to study the verbal behavior of humans, you've got to use a standardized way of eliciting the speech. So we developed a standardized way of eliciting speech and these are the instructions. "This is a microphone here. This is a study of speaking and conversational habits. I would like you to talk for five minutes about any interesting or dramatic personal life experiences you've ever had. While you're talking, I would prefer not to reply to any questions you might have until the five minutes is over. You can talk about one experience and if the five minutes is not over, you can talk about another. Do you have any questions now?" The subject might ask what is interesting or dramatic? If the subject does, the answer is: "I don't know what's interesting and dramatic as far as you're concerned." And you can say, "Don't worry about me, just whatever you think", Yes, purposely turning the question back to the speaker. "Do you have any questions now?" If the subject says that he/she does not, then the interviewer says. "Alright you can start now and, then, five minutes later, I will tell you to stop." Now, that situation, we studied it very carefully. To get a reliable sample, a person has to speak at least eighty- five words. If they speak less in that five minute period, the sample isn't good enough, just like getting a blood sample, you know, if the sample is too small for some tests the results may not be acceptably reliable. As you know, you now can do a good job with very tiny amounts of blood these day, but for our content analysis measure, you need that much, a minimum of 85 words. Those speech samples are recorded and the typescript is typed, at this stage, in text or ASCII or word perfect 5.1, (and lately in Microsoft Word) because the program, the artificial intelligence software program, it's called LISP, is programmed to understand the above computer programs. Now, the way they scored, the software program, when it is typed up, it's going to get ordinary punctuation. Its periods may be commas. It depends on the secretary. And, the program needs help; you might have a compound sentence, so it might be separated by a comma. So, the typist has to put in a slash or diagonal and that tells it that a clause has occurred (Now our software program recognizes and does all this clausing by itself.). Now, to get an answer to the key question. What do you examine there? Well, the program understands all parsing. What's parsing? Parsing is a capacity to label each part of speech, noun, pronoun, adjective, verb, adverb, preposition, conjunction, and so on. All that information, over two hundred thousand words, has been put in the computer and the computer knows these data. Now, we could have a program to do that, to teach it. It knows that a word like "hide" can be a verb or it can be a noun, so it has that already. So, what does that tell us to do? Well, it can tell, it knows the parts of speech; it understands that there's a difference between, "He hit me" and "I hit myself". And, that makes a difference in psychiatry, you know, about whether you're going to conclude, "I like myself" or "I hate myself" or "Somebody doesn't like me". Now, in addition to having the knowledge, the semantic knowledge of every, over two hundred thousand words (or idiomatic phrases), it is informed about every slang expression, so if somebody says, "I kick the bucket", usually, that doesn't mean somebody went and kicked a bucket, it means somebody is going to die, or did die, or will die, or I die. And, so, it has in its dictionary every slang expression that one can think of. Now, you're going to say, "Well, gee, how can it have every possible one"? Well, we just keep adding to the computer programs dictionary, because we hear another common word or expression that merits addition to the computer program's memory. You know, like the word, "it sucks". Well, gee, I mean, under certain circumstances that means something isn't good, but if you say, "the baby sucks", well, that's a problem. Even, then, there's some ambiguity, so with this program, what it's doing, now to get to your question, it's taken me two minutes already, it first searches out the meanings of the words, does probably what humans do; it first goes through every word and expression and it has in its memory that could fit into the anxiety scale. The anxiety scale is divided up into six sub-scales: death, mutilation, separation, guilt, shame and diffuse anxiety. An example of diffuse anxiety = I'm nervous and I feel guilty is guilt anxiety, and I was embarrassed is shame anxiety. Now, the computer dictionary has somebody, mainly myself, classify every word, how it can be used. I may miss some, possibly have, but the computer, if it makes an error, at least, in contrast to you and me, it's consistent, keeps making the same error. You know, it's programmed just a certain way and some it doesn't know. And, so, the first thing it does, it searches all this. It's hard for me to empathize with it because it's going so fast as electricity. It goes through all these words, every dot, and it says, well, this might be classified, because this word could be classified in several scales and it registers inside of it. I'm trying to read its mind. It says, well, this could be a candidate for this score or that score. Now, it searches more about who did what to whom, because that makes a difference. I don't whether I do that in fact or not, but this is the way we worked out and taught the computer. And, so, it registers all these candidates and, then, when it decides, well this is the most possible, the most likely, it suggests, inside of it, this score be classified. Now, it takes that score and, now, compares that, it adds, tallies, that score to all the other instances and candidates, because somebody could, both, talking as I am, could both say something that is hostile to others and hostile to oneself. You know, "I shot myself in the foot and, also, him". And, so, people would say all kinds of things. So, it may score some verbal statements on several scales and it adds all those up. Now, it compares those to norms. Now, where did it get the norms? Well, we got thousands of verbal samples on people that seemed to fall under the norms. At least, they're working and mentally and physically healthy. And, now, it should adjust those norms to the educational level. After all, if you have a verbal sample from a five-year-old kid and something from a college graduate from Princeton, well, you know, they're going to be some differences with respect to cognitive function, according to age and educational level. So, the software program makes some adjustments for that. By then, it asks how many standard deviations is this verbal sample, with all the scores summed up, according to the weights on these scales, different from the norms, one, two or three standard deviations and it tells you that. Now, if you want to go further, if you want it to, on this, the basis of applied in a verbal sentence, after a statement of disclaimers program so we don't get sued and say, you know, this is only five minute verbal sample. It's more reliable the more words you have, but it says the clinician might consider these diagnostic classifications from the Diagnostic Statistical Manual (DSM-IV) of the American Psychiatric Association. That wasn't a very good summary on my part, but it gives you a general idea of how the software works.

TB: It's an excellent summary, a logical process, really.

LG: Gradually, it aims to be logical.

TB: Gradually.

LG: Now, that's the way it goes. Now, it comes up with those scores and we, even, used (I've been checking on the way here) years back (If you live long enough you can do a lot of studies); I've lived pretty long. We did earlier studies, years back, when we had a NIAAA Alcoholism Research Center, we looked at, could five-minute verbal samples, just taking pieces of the scores, how well can we develop regression formulas that tell you or predict neuropsychological test scores from the Halstead-Reitan Cognitive tests. We keep trying mathematics again. And we found some regression formulas that, to a level of .01 or .001, predict Halsted-Reitan Categories tests, and all you need to do that is a five-minute verbal sample. And, we use that. The program will print that out if the cognitive impairment score is more than one standard deviation from the norm, it prints out all these regression formulas. Well, I haven't replicated that. Just lately, on this last study here, I've given you a reprint on it. From those data, I'm seeing how well as I replicated. After all, you can get different samples, but the system is pretty good. So, that's about how it goes.

TB: Well, that is, actually, you gave us the necessary information, because when we get back to it, we'll know now what we are talking about. Let me just go for a second, from Cincinnati, you were in Cincinnati until?

LG: 1967.

TB: '67. Then, you moved to Irvine, as the founding Chair and you stayed in Irvine, actually, after serving, I don't know many years.

LG: Well, I came to UCI in 1967, and, then I was Chair for about twelve years and became head of the Psychiatric Counsult and Liaison Service at the UCI Medical Center. I did that for a while and, then, I became the Scientific Co-director of an Alcoholism Research Center funded by the National Institute of Alcohol and Alcohol Abuse (NIAAA) and that Center was composed of a conglomerate of basic scientists and clinical scientists. And what was the main theme of our Research Center? The Effect of Alcohol on the Nervous System. We were looking at humans and looking at sub-human animals and we had some powerful research people from molecular biology and from neurobiology, and we worked together for about 10 years.

TB: The Center for Alcohol Research, I suppose.

LG: And that Center turned out to be relevant to looking and getting more data on cognitive impairment function.

TB: So, basically, when you retired from the Department of Psychiatry Chairmanship, right, then, you built this other Institute. You, also, became Professor of Sociology and Ecology. Am I correct?

LG: Social Ecology and Social Science. Even when I was Chairman of Psychiatry, though I had courtesy appointments there, because it was useful. I mean, you know, in a research University in the University of California system, it is useful and productive to get cross fertilized and work in several departments.

TB: How long did you direct, actually, the Institute, the other Institute?

LG: Well, the grant lasted for about eight or nine years.

TB: When was that with Irvine?

LG: I don't know, precisely.

TB: Approximately? In the eighties?

LG: Probably, yes it was into the eighties.

TB: Into the eighties, mid-eighties or something like that, right? And, after then, you just moved back to the Department of Psychiatry and Human Behavior?

LG: Well, I was in that Department all the time.

TB: All the time?

LG: All the time, yes.

TB: And, you are still actively working, right? And, what are you working on now?

LG: I'm still in the Department, Professor Emeritus, and I'm working full-time and I see patients, maybe fifteen to twenty hours a week, maybe ten to fifteen hours a week, children and adults. I continue to do research and I do writing. And, I have a research grant. I'm funded right now for a research project from NIDA, the National Institute on Drug Abuse.

TB: So, you still have, actually, a grant, ongoing grant?

LG: Ongoing grant and I collaborate with one of the younger professors, Jerry McGuire, who is Director of Geriatrics and who has drug grants and, so, we're getting verbal samples on some of those patients, drug grants for Alzheimer's drugs.

TB: Maybe we should have five minutes to have something. Is that alright?

LG: Sure.

TB: And, then, we continue for another forty-five. Would you like us to go? We can go.

So, you moved in 1953 to Cincinnati and around that time chlorpromazine comes in, chlorpromazine and reserpine just comes in while you were in Cincinnati. Then, in 1957, imipramine, so the antidepressants are coming in. And, actually, meprobamate is already around. Then, in 1960, the benzodiazipines are coming along, and they do lean to the spirit. You are becoming interested in psychopharmacology. By that time, there is a change in the structure of psychiatry, very rapidly, sort of from hospitalized inpatient to outpatient psychiatry. So, all of this is taking place, really, during the time you were in Cincinnati and like, in everything, you pick up things at the very early kind of stage. Should you become interested in psychopharmacology? And, maybe if you could just elaborate a little bit to see what did you do, even, the different areas in which you become involved, because you had been involved through psychosomatics, but, then, you could, also, very early, you became involved in pharmacokinetics and so on, so maybe if you could just elaborate, how you got involved in psychopharmacology.

LG: Well, I could say it just happened, but, usually things happen for a reason. I was, naturally, awfully interested in the major tranquilizers, since the chlorpromazines, they had remarkable effects on patients. There were some patients we saw in Fort Worth, Texas from

World War I, I mean World War II. I did have a group of three hundred patients that were assigned to me from World War I. That's why I included that. They were moved from St. Elizabeth's mental hospital in Washington, D.C. to under my care, also, at Fort Worth. But, in any case, the main drugs we had in Fort Worth were apomorphine and hyoscine, to try to deal with very belligerent and violent patients (which made these inpatients nauseated and likely to vomit) or electro shock therapy; so this, actually, I was quite interested in that and the thorazine and, also, some of the other medication like the benzodiazipines. And, I found, that in developing these content analysis scales, I thought, well here's a medication that content analysis scales should be relevant to and, if, indeed, the criteria I used to validate the content analysis scales that I'd developed were valid. I'd, not only, used psychological measures that are used in the judgment of psychiatrists listening to patients but biochemical measures, that is, if there's changes in pro plasma free fatty acids of individuals, fasting, that might be an indicator, a biochemical indicator of adrenergic impulses and, also, what better than to see what kind of anti-anxiety drug does it effect these scales.

TB: May I just....you mentioned hyoscine and apomorphine. It seems to be that you are still someone like myself, because we use hyoscine and apomorphine. Have you ever used tincture of opium, as well, in depression?

LG: No.

TB: So, you really just have, correct, controlling excitement?

LG: I'm not even sure that you can get tincture of opium in the United States.

TB: No, no, it was around, yes, when I went to (inaudible). They knew about it. I have a feeling they used it.

LG: Is that right?

TB: Yes, yes, this was sort of in the early fifties, I guess.

LG: Where was this that you could get it?

TB: Well, actually, I definitely remembering using it in Hungary, but if my recollection is correct, when I arrived to Montreal, which was in '57, it was just about the time when Heinz Lehmann published the first paper on this side of the Atlantic on librium. It was just one year, a little bit after, when he presented his first paper and we talked about it, what they used before, and if my recollection is correct, he mentioned that they used tincture of opium.

LG: But, in Canada, but not in the United States.

TB: In Canada.

LG: That's what I mean.

TB: Are you sure?

LG: I think not in the United States.

TB: I don't know.

LG: What morphine and heroin are derivatives of?

TB: That's what they used. I have seen apomorphine used. In Hungary we also used morphine. Anyway, we used that, used propanaldehyde.

LG: Chloral hydrate?

TB: Chloral hydrate and bromides.

LG: Bromides. Some people can get bromide intoxication.

TB: Yes. And, during the period, you see, it was just a period when you started, when neurosyphilis became eradicated, to some extent, especially, in the United States where you live. Actually, pellagra had just wiped out, to some extent, right? But, anyway, you had experience with it and you mentioned that when chlorpromazine came, you immediately picked it up, right?

LG: A magic drug.

TB: Magic. How did you feel about it?

LG: Well, very enthusiastic, yes. But, it was true that it worked and it really did.

TB: But, you, really, did not do any work with it, basically?

LG: Oh, yes. I didn't publish, but I was a psychiatrist at Cincinnati General. We used it. As I was saying, it worked.

TB: It worked. What about reserpine? Did you have any experience?

LG: Yes, we used it some, sure.

TB: But, then reserpine, also. What about meprobamate?

LG: Oh, yes. All of these.

LG: We had some patients, later, that became addicted to meprobamate and, then, you know, when you withdraw meprobamate some patients are going to have seizures.

TB: And, so, you really worked with all....

LG: I was on a busy clinical service, you know.

TB: Really, the first research, really, what you did in psychopharmacology, I'm not talking about biochemical measures, you know, linking to psychosomatic kind of work, which was the drug you worked with besides pipradrol?.

LG: I don't remember exactly, but there are drugs like the benzodiazepines and perphenazine.

TB: Perphenazine is the first publication, I noticed, you see. Could you just, a little bit, elaborate. What did you do, you know?

LG: Oh, yes. We had a busy clinical service for a number of patients, who were put on perphenazine. And I wanted to see, did the content analysis scales I was developing, hostility scales around that time, work well and usefully? These were content analysis scales that measure three types of hostility: hostility outward, hostility inward, and ambivalent hostility and in these patients, did the perphenazine effect the scores in the hostility scales? And they did. They suppressed all three types of hostility. So, that's how I happened to get into that.

TB: I kind of forced this perphenazine issue, now. What the perphenazine, actually, besides pipradrol, was this the first sort of psychopharmacology oriented research?

LG: Tom, I don't think that way, because, I mean, I feel like I'm on a witness stand. I don't think of whether or not I was first It was one of the many studies, actually, I was involved in. It seems to be, some early benzodiazipine study about the same time. But, I'd have to look over my CV. I don't try to memorize the order of my publications.

TB: No, no, no, it's unimportant.

LG: I don't want to fail on this test you're giving me. I want to get a good grade.

TB: With that, you could only pass with flying.colors. No. Actually, it seems to be that you worked with several things, simultaneously, right? And, probably in several ways. With perphenazine, you were really interested in hostility, mainly, and what about the benzodiazipine?

LG: Yes, I was interested in the benzodiazipine and at that stage, chlordiazpoxide.

TB: Chlordiazpoxide?.

LG: And I wanted to find out whether these scales were any good, you know. The chlordiazpoxide should lower the anxiety scale scores, you know, significantly, as compared to a placebo. And, I got into the studies like that, testing out, to see whether the methodology was really good—a form of construct validation. I mean, the content scales were, you know, the major focus and not testing the drug as much as the scales. Do they really measure? Because, I was into the validity of any measurement procedure. So, that was one. But, I certainly was interested in librium, (chlordiazpoxide) and all the other benzodiazipine derivatives, as I reflect on it now. Then, I, later, did studies with valium (diazepam) and lorazepam, you know, an ativan and many of the other benzodiazepines, such as, triazolam.

TB: So, you went with triazolam in sleep or?

LG: No, no.

TB: Just in general?

LG: No, generally, to see what, if any, effect it'd have on the scores of the content analysis scales.

TB: So, you really...

LG: And, what was the relationship of these psychoactive medications, to even the pharmacokinetics, the blood levels, to the magnitude of the psychobiological effect that they might have on the scale measures. And, I found out the content analysis scales were, indeed, capable of measuring what they were purported to measure.

TB: So, really, you were interested in the scales, not just in yours, but you were also interested in developing your scales, prominently, but, at the same time, you were interested in all kinds of scales, what they are able to do, how the drugs effect the scores on the scales, right? And you say that approach is referred to as construct validation?

LG: Exactly.

TB: And, you had been involved with, it seems to be, with a number of neuroleptics like perphenazine. I have a feeling thioridazine and some of the others, later.

LG: Later. Then, I got involved and I had some funded grants on that. Looking at that was, I think that was more in California, on thioridazine and mesoridazine, to see whether they made any difference on the effects and, also, the pharmacokinetics.

I compared the pharmacokinetics and, then, I got into the metabolites in thioridazine. And, I'll mention, before I forget it, I think it's an area that's still neglected. I detected that one of the metabolites of thioridazine, it was sulforidazine or a sulfoxide that was probably responsible for the adverse effects that some people get on cardiovascular function with test drugs. And, I tried to get a lot of that sulforidazine or sulfoxide from Sandoz (the pharmaceutical company that made these drugs), and they were interested in the paper. They, actually, gave me some money, voluntarily, to study thioridazine, but when I said I wanted to study it further and find out, because I could reduce the amount of that thioridazine or sulfoxide so people wouldn't have that adverse effect, they didn't want to fund it. I suppose now, I don't like to go down in history now, but they were doing alright with thioridazine, and they didn't want to fool around with that aspect of its clinical usefulness.

TB: No, I think it is perfectly alright. We should talk about it. I think it is really very important because it happens to be that thioridazine was the first neuroleptic, in which the prolongation of QT interval on the EKG, was brought to attention. I have a feeling that a few people died, if my recollection is correct, it was in Kingston, Ontario and it was very carefully observed.

LG: Is that right?

TB: Yes, it was quite carefully followed up, especially, the control studies.

LG: Why didn't Sandoz want to help fund it?

TB: I don't know, but you certainly made an important contribution, because through your interest in pharmacokinetics, you picked up that, probably, the sulfoxide metabolite is responsible and made a contribution.

LG: The drug's possibly adverse effect kept me interested. Everybody else said, well, that metabolite is not pharmacologically active. Now, it doesn't have any effect on the psychosis but it has another biological effect. And, what I'm saying. And now in trying to get the head of the organic chemistry department at UCI, I asked her whether she could manufacture the metabolite, and they could for a certain amount of money, because I wanted to test the effects of the metabolite on cardiovascular function in dog experiments. But, I never was able to obtain the necessary funds. The point I want to make is, I think, in general, pharmaceutical companies are not very interested in trying to discover more concerning what triggers the adverse side effects of drugs. And I was interested and I still am. And, I think it's a neglected research area, because I think it's possible, with other medications, to avoid those adverse side effects. But the drug companies don't seem to be interested.

TB: But, actually, you are, I think the matter is very, very important. You contributed a bit. How did you, actually, happen to think that it was that metabolite of thioridazine, which is capable of causing a prolongation of QT, actually, which can cause ventricular fibrillation and it can, actually, lead to death, a very dangerous metabolite and it happens within the administration of thioridazine, right? Anyway, how did you pick that metabolite?

LG: We were getting, we got regular blood levels from the patients that were getting thioridazine and we got, not only, the blood levels of thioridazine but all the metabolites. And, then, we would get EKG's on the patients and, then, we'd look at those patients that had higher levels of that metabolite. As you probably know, not everybody metabolizes these medications the same way, and we picked the patients that had the higher levels of the metabolite at the time they were having their abnormal EKG.

TB: Did you do just one speed or speed it up, because sometimes it's easier to conduct this type. Anyway, I just wondered. You can't pick it up in a normal EKG, but, you know, really.

LG: Well, first of all, we had the means and we had the equipment and I was into that kind of research, then, and I had a lab at that time to enable me to look at the matter. It was more a focus on the metabolites.

TB: Metabolites, right?

LG: And, we discovered, I didn't keep following that, but we discovered some metabolites in some of the drugs, I notice in just looking over my CV, that other people never reported. Well, that got me pretty far off the main direction of my research, at this point, but I had a young collaborator, Eugene Dinovo, who was out of UCLA and he loved doing that kind of research. We had a great time collaborating together. I think that's not a bad way to go. There should be more studies. It's an open field, the study of adverse side effects of drugs and metabolites. People don't look into that.

TB: Is there any other research you did besides the research that detected the sulfoxide? Is there any other what you linked to an adverse side effect? I mean, because this is an important one line of research.

LG: Oh, I think it's important. I'm just thinking. No, but I do remember that Eugene really enjoyed working with me. I'm going to regress, momentarily, just to let people know years from now, that we had our problems funding research. He was a bench researcher. He was on soft money, you know. I had to keep getting grants to fund him. And, he had a family and was brilliant. He, later, got a position and is probably still working at it, as Director of the Pathology Lab at one of the VA Hospitals, but we, together, discovered some other metabolites that were not in the scientific literature. But we didn't try to see whether they were related to anything, because we didn't have the funds. You know, when you have these federal grants, you can look at certain things, but you can't go too far off, because you've got a public responsibility to focus on the principal goals of your research.

TB: So, you really.

LG: There may be others, but we discovered, I think, that some of those other metabolites might be related to adverse symptoms.

TB: But, it was not followed up, because of the soft money, right? So, you're really trying to bring to our attention that the grant system is very good, but it could be better.

LG: Oh, yes. It should have been, and, then, you have to carry on in the same way. You decide what your priorities are. I tend to want to pursue a lot of interesting things, but I have to say, think. You have to think, what's the first priority?

TB: Well, anyway, you made a major discovery, because you linked a side effect to a metabolite, which, you really think, it should have been followed up more properly, but.....

LG: I think, I'm right, not only there, but Sandoz, I visited them a couple of times there in Basel. I'm sure that their higher ups just advised them not to spend money on that line of research, and they were doing alright on the drug, but, you know, I still think that's a hot tip. For anybody else, I don't think, in general, you can get the pharmaceutical company to want to invest what triggers some of the adverse side effects. I may be wrong.

TB: So, this is interviewing you are wouldn't like to go too far with it; it just happens to be that we were the first ones. I published the first control study about this part of side effects. It just happens.

LG: Oh, you did! I didn't know that.

TB: It just happens to be and I was very much involved with the same people and I got exactly the same condition.

LG: Fascinating.

TB: So, let's just get a little bit, maybe, we are in the mid-sixties at this point. But, I, also, learned something else from you, that you tried to use this test, primarily your own test, than all other different tests to discriminate among the drugs. You mentioned that one thing was the metabolites. You tried to pick up side effects, but, you, also, am I correct, you, also, mentioned you tried to see the differences. Did you or did I misunderstand? Can you, would you like to elaborate?

LG: The difference is between drugs.

TB: Just picking it up through the different tests. Or, you didn't say that. I had the feeling that you were doing something with the speech analysis, trying to see if there were any differences between thioridazine and perphenazine or mesoridazine.

LG: No, I didn't.

TB: You didn't do that?

LG: No.

TB: You were mainly in pharmacokinetics and, then, you, also, started a very early kind of state, biochemical and of kinetics like you already mentioned, when you were director, you worked, I think, with hypertension. Would you like to just elaborate?

LG: I studied the effect of hydrochlorothiazide on hypertensives and did it affect, the hydrochlorothiazide, did it affect, not only the blood pressure, but did it have an effect on the subjects' language? And, it did.

TB: Did it correlate with the therapeutic effect or correlate it with the?

LG: Yes.

TB: So, it did. So, you could pick it up through the language, as well as from the blood pressure measurement.

LG: As well, as the blood pressure.

TB: So, thank you very much. I think we probably ran out of tape.

TB: We are continuing the interview with Dr. Gottschalk. We are in the 1960's. He is working in Cincinnati and he has become involved in psychopharmacology. He did, already, some important work with thioridazine and identifying certain metabolites and we will be continuing the discussion with some of the work he did with hydrochlorothiazide in hypertension, which he correlated to therapeutic effect in hypertension, with content analysis of speech. At all the same time, he was, also, involved in some biochemical measures and maybe this is where we should pick it up. If you could, just elaborate a little bit what you have done.

LG: Well, around that time, Tom, more and more convincing, we had a useful and valuable measure in the content analysis measure of anxiety and hostility. And I thought I'd like to validate it some more, with respect to a combination of biochemical factors and physiological associations, such as, the measure in the blood streams of subjects. At that time, there was not a good measure of adrenergic substances such as epinephrine and norepinephrine, which was thought to be involved in influencing the magnitude of states of anxiety or hostility. There are such measures now, but at that time, there was one measure, fasting plasma-free fatty acids, and plasma-free fatty acids. These are released from the liver and fat storages in response to a chemical substance that's secreted in the blood stream and in association with the arousal of anxiety or fear or anger. And, so, I decided to use that measure, namely, plasma-free fatty acids, and we did a number of measures showing that (and these appeared in published papers) showed that the higher the anxiety levels in individuals, normal individuals, the higher the plasma-free fatty acids, which demonstrated to our satisfaction that this thing we're measuring from language, this construct, anxiety or fear, is biologically associated with the arousal of adrenergic substances. We did a lot of other studies using that. As I said, it was the only measure in those times that was available. And, we noted subsequently that if you drew blood from a subject where you're getting a five minute speech sample, and you drew blood before and after the end of five-minutes, the free fatty acids went higher in those people, the more anxious they were during that five minutes. And, we, also, noted that in dreaming subjects, if you drew blood from them during rapid eye movement sleep, at the beginning of rapid eye movement sleep, and fifteen minutes later, for measurement of plasma-free fatty acids and, then, had them report their dream and, then, you scored the dream on my anxiety scale for anxiety, the higher the anxiety in the dream scored, the higher the free fatty acids went, while the patient was dreaming, without reporting the dream, just dreaming about it. And, that article was published in Science and I think it had an interesting effect. It means that without talking about anxiety, just seeing visual pictures in which appears there's more anxiety than some other person's dream, the more arousal of adrenergic substances. I had an interesting query in answer to that paper from a number of people. Scientists writing, "if there's more anxiety in dreams, there's more arousal of adrenergic substances and in some instances that could be fatal, just from a dream." I thought this was an amusing query. I was asked "Why not recommend that everybody get psychoanalyzed and that might put an end to anxiety dreams?" And, I had to write them, that doesn't put an end to anxiety dreams. A person may still have anxiety and they might understand better what the anxiety is about in the dream. And, so much for those studies, it seems.

TB: You certainly correlated anxiety with plasma-free fatty acid levels.

LG: Well, and, presumably, I wasn't interested in merely plasma-free fatty acids. But more that there was some psychosomatic relevance with respect to cholesterol or fatty acid problems. And it corroborated our impression that this dimension measured from language was associated with physiological and neurobiological and biochemical concomitants in the body and wasn't just a matter of the mind. It was the speech and what was said and its semantics that involved the brain and the whole body.

TB: And, really, the test picked it up?

LG: Right.

TB: You know, it correlated it very highly.

LG: I think there's, when you ask me these matters, I get a flood of remembrances. We noted that people in Cincinnati that were into sports, had all around lower plasma-free fatty acids, than people who were not involved in sports. That kind of finding might support what's talked about a lot now, especially in California, but probably in the great state of Tennessee or in Canada, Toronto, that a certain amount of exercise is pretty good for the body, as well as for the mind. I do recommend to a patient once in awhile, "Healthy Body, Healthy Mind."

There's something to it. Is there anything else? Yes, we looked at, not only, plasma-free fatty acids, but blood cholesterol. And there's no paper labeling that, but we did find that the higher the hostility scores, the greater the blood cholesterol in normal subjects and I don't think that's been made a lot of these days. But there certainly is a lot of preoccupation these day with elevated cholesterol. In those days, back there in the sixties, we didn't take a look at whether this was a LDH or high HDL cholesterol. We weren't taking a look. We were just getting total cholesterols. I don't think clinicians were thinking about those things. But, it's an interesting finding and, also, triglycerides, nowadays, where I am now. I sometimes get triglycerides on individuals.

TB: So, you really were very much involved in cholesterol, free fatty acid and triglycerides. You did make all the special tests?

LG: Oh, yes, triglycerides, cholesterol and so on. That was probably part of the influence of being in that Cincinnati environment. As I say, it was pretty psychosomatic, but we were looking, secondarily, at what do these emotions that people carry around with them, what effect, if any, does that have on the fatty acid and triglyceride metabolism? It probably does have some. I haven't gotten back, and that was a Cincinnati period, I haven't gotten back into that, but I noticed that in the current literature, there's some interest.

TB: Oh, yes, there's interest for permanently now. Actually, you see, you did a local correlation, actually, with anxiety, hostility and free fatty acid, this type of thing. Going back just a little bit, which you already talked about, we talked about that you worked quite a bit with benzodiazepines, with benzodiazepines in metabolism and your instrument and you worked, also, in relation to hostility. Is there anything special that you picked up in the relationship to benzodiazepines and hostility?

LG: I was telling, a hostility outward score is, to some extent, also, decreased by the benzodiazepines.

TB: Well, that's really what you found?

LG: Yes, we found that.

TB: Now, we are, also, in this area of anxiety and did you work, besides with benzodiazepines, like beta blockers, propranolol?

LG: Yes, we worked with them.

TB: You did some work with them?

LG: And, we found, in one of the papers, one of the reports and studies, that in relatively normal individuals the beta blocker, also, significantly, reduced anxiety levels, using this verbal sample approach, and I tried to get into rather old psychophysiological relationship as, (let's see what I can recall) whether people get anxious because of changes in the peripheral nervous system or is it primarily a central brain phenomenon? There were old theories about that.

TB: Did you work with James Lang?

LG: James Lang, that's right. Thanks for reminding me. And, I didn't study on that.

TB: What did you find?

LG: I didn't study on that and publish it. What did I find? Apparently, it attracted a lot of attention, but I found that beta blockers do, indeed, decrease anxiety levels on my scales, content analysis scales, but the plasma-free fatty acids, fasting plasma-free fatty acids, were not significant, they were decreased, but not significantly.

TB: I see.

LG: And, I concluded, since I was seeing the plasma-free fatty acid responses, partly a measure of peripheral nervous system, autonomic nervous system, can't be sure of that, but that was more a measure of that, because we were using a beta blocker.

And, there are other beta blockers that go through blood brain barriers, but I made a point that this was primarily, I was just using that beta blocker that anxiety we were measuring was primarily a central nervous system phenomena, but it didn't prove that it couldn't be peripheral. There's other studies that we did that demonstrated, what most of us already know, that if your heartbeat is faster, I think this involved, this was studied using benzodiazepines, if you're, that the autonomic nervous system reinforcement of anxiety enhances or increases the anxiety and, so, you know, when I give patients, today, benzodiazepine and they have panic disorder, I think, well, they don't get that feedback from an increased heart rate and so on. It works to some extent. But, anyway, that paper, published at that time, attracted the attention, apparently, of a large German company like Bayer, and I was invited, this was a marvelous experience, once in awhile, there's a payoff in science, to an international meeting of cardiologists in Venice, where I presented that paper, because the cardiologists were quite interested in these details. Later, I published, I think it's a book chapter, a chapter on beta blockers and the different kinds. So, again, in that case, the non-psychiatrists, the cardiologists were quite interested in that research and finding. I don't know that I answered all the questions in my mind. But, there weren't any better measures at that time for measuring adrenaline and noradrenaline in the peripheral nervous system.

TB: Actually, you made some important contributions, again, like with thioridazine. Because you seem to have separated these benzodiazepiness and with propranolol, two different kind of anxiety. You kind of have one, which is central, because even if it is controlled, the free fatty acids are not changing. Am I right? If it's correctly controlled, then, the other anxiety and free fatty acids go hand in hand and your speech analysis can pick up both. And, I don't think that you go beyond that trying to characterize the two different kinds of anxieties, but I don't think you want to.

LG: Well, I don't know the anxieties are any different.

TB: Any different.

LG: I don't think the phenomenon we measure with my content analysis measure differentiates, as a matter of fact, anxiety, which is sometimes called "neurotic fear," from "genuine fear." So, as that measure is concerned, it's measuring arousal whether it is neurotic or real fear. There really is a line there, that somebody is going to kill you. It doesn't differentiate.

TB: It really doesn't differentiate. It just measures anxiety.

LG: Anxiety fear.

TB: Right. And, again, this is probably the kinds of things you did in the area of anxiety, right? Or, did you do any other work in this particular area?

LG: Well, I think the major tranquilizers, also, reduce anxiety, too, you know, they, so to speak, knock somebody out. And, for that matter, as you suggested before here, briefly and privately, the opium, tincture of opium, an opiate derivative, demerol meperidine, also reduces anxiety and hostility and the amount of reduction is related to the blood level. So, those are other studies we did.

TB: But, you, actually, published on that, yes. So, this was, more or less, the field of anxiety and it looks like that you did some work again in pharmacokinetics, some other work with different drugs, other than the methazines, right, thioridazine and a number of other methazines, am I correct?

LG: I'm sorry, I didn't.

TB: You did some pharmacokinetic work, not only thioridazine. You did with a number of different drugs. Now, did you do your neuroleptic in Cincinnati in the 1960's. You did some work on neuroleptic withdrawal, with some chronic hospitalized mental patients.

LG: Yes, in Cincinnati.

TB: Cincinnati.

LG: That way, we were able to, somehow it was really difficult to achieve, at the Longview State Mental Hospital, which had a lot of chronic schizophrenics. I got the hunch that some of those schizophrenics seemed pretty normal to me, I mean, by this time, after they had been there about ten years. And, there was an issue about whether or not, I think it was beginning to appear, there could be adverse effects on patients on chronic administration of phenothiazines. What if we discontinued the phenothiazines on a group, a large group of patients, seventy-five; we had to certainly alert the staff, get the hospital cooperation. I could convince, in some way, you've got a lot of patients here. You may not have to have them here any more. But, there are other things that might be, say, and, anyway, we did that study and we did find that a certain number of patients, maybe a third or a half, remained about the same or seemed even better, more collaborative. At that time, I was developing a scale for measurement of the magnitude or severity of schizophrenia and the scale, I named it, Social Alienation-Personal Disorganization Scale. And, we got those measures on these patients before and after withdrawal of the large amount of phenothiazines that were on. They were on different phenothiazines. I found out that those inpatients in whom the social alienation-personal disorganization (SAPD) score before taking them off the phenothiazine was one that would probably be okay if you discontinued their medication. And those patients whose

SAPD scores were well above that, they tended to go up, get worse, very significantly. And it was, I think, of considerable interest at that time. It demonstrated that not all chronic schizophrenic patients had to be, for the rest of their lives, kept on a major tranquilizer. The drugs could probably be used that way. And so, we discontinued this practice. And, a fair number of patients though they were off such medication for a while, they were able to be discharged from the hospital.

TB: So, really, you had a demonstration that maybe as high as fifty percent probably did not need to be kept on their medication. So there was, really, a significant finding. In the maintenance of psychoactive medication or prophylaxis--whatever you would like to call it—a psychiatric patient's drug treatment should be individualized rather than following a generalized formula.

LG: Exactly. You're right there. There are either different kinds of schizophrenia or different types of severity. I am going to slide back to my days of Public Health Service Hospital in Ft. Worth, Texas, because I kept up with my caseload. It was a terribly heavy caseload, but I was awarded by the Public Health Service with responsibility for three hundred patients. Over three hundred patients had been moved from St. Elizabeth's Hospital in Washington, D.C., and they were from World War I and they were transferred to the USPHS hospital in Fort Worth. First, they weren't getting any medications. By this time, you know, twenty, maybe twenty-five or more years after they'd had "shell shock" or a nervous breakdown or whatever, many of them were in good shape. They were schizophrenic, but now they had various medical problems, which was an interesting experience on patients that are hospitalized for a long, long time, pretty healthy. So, that, I'd often wondered now, some of those, if I asked them, you know, did they remember much about their experience, because they had not received shock treatment. They were unspoiled patients, had not had shock treatment, probably not hyoscine and apomorphine. It was very difficult, by the way, to find their relatives and so on. And, I tried to, in my spare time, which I didn't have much, see where I could discharge home, some. But, I just wondered whether most of them, I would say hadn't recovered, but were in pretty good shape. Some of them, by this time, had organic disabilities or had other kinds of problems.

TB: Let's go back to this cohort of schizophrenics at Longview State Hospital in Cincinnati. The number, which was seventy to a hundred, right, around seventy patients, whom you took off, right, medication.

LG: Oh, yes, seventy-five.

TB: Seventy-five people. This is a very important and interesting topic. Your listed implications are far reaching, like how did you take them off? Did you go cold turkey or gradually reduce the medication?

LG: We cold turkeyed them, but we substituted their psychoactive medication with a placebo. And because it's not that easy to do, because the hospital personnel, especially the nursing staff didn't want it done.

TB: But anyway, you took them completely off.

LG: So, placebo was studied now. It was cold turkey.

TB: Cold turkey placebo. Was there any withdrawal effect?

LG: Not at that time.

TB: Now, it seems to be, you tried to really identify who are those who need phenothiazine or neuroleptics and where are the ones who did not. And, again, in your characteristic and usual way, you did not go to try to figure out whether methodology or psychopathology could help, but you developed your own instrument. Are there any additions to it?

LG: Well, the common denominator for all these patients, in terms of psychopathology, is that they were all schizophrenics, chronic or undifferentiated; so, in that sense, from the viewpoint of nomenclature, they were the same, rather than random.

TB: Yes, but some people.....

LG: That was the only thing.

TB: You took them as chronic and differentiated.

LG: That's right.

TB: And, you really developed, did you develop this social alienation-personal disorganization scale?

LG: Yes.

TB: You did?

LG: There are a number of papers on that content analysis scale.

TB: Your contribution, again, there is a relationship with the level of disorganization; right, the more disorganized the more they are in need of neuroleptics, right?

LG: Yes. If somebody, in giving a five-minute verbal sample and did blocking or started the sentence and didn't finish it and blocked, that was scored. It's not just content, but form of speech. And if they made bizarre statements, you know, like "I saw somebody walking on the ceiling last night", you know, other bizarre things, or showed paranoid tendencies articulated in their speech, these verbal data would also be scored on that scale, similarly to the verbal items that trained psychiatrists typically use to make a diagnosis of schizophrenia. In contrast to the diagnosis of depressive disorders or affective disorders, which may have delusions. So, that's what that scale, the SAPD scale, incorporated. Now, it overlapped, later, with another scale that we developed for depression. After all, some people with bad depressions can be delusional and have somatic delusions and so on. It's not hard to do. What psychiatrists, typically and regularly use as a major criteria for deciding somebody's schizophrenia, especially, the thought disorder, they measure.

TB: Was it, primarily, what people would call today, the positive symptoms or was it really positive and negative, with, you know, somebody who is inaccessible, inappropriate, in an emotional score?

LG: Well, to the extent that such a distinction can be identified in language; somebody would have to say, in terms of negative symptoms, "Well, I sleep all of the time", or "I don't have any energy". They'd have to make a statement along that line. Now, I can't say, because I haven't, I wouldn't say cared about, but I've thought about it some, but I don't know that it's crucial. In those days that we were doing that, there wasn't this big distinction between positive and negative symptoms and I'm not absolutely convinced they are that important, but it looks like there may be some difference. Well, I'm just thinking about something. I'm trying to explain why I didn't and I think that, you asked me, and I think there are some, my scales could probably be broken down to differentiate between positive and negative symptoms, but I have to work on that.

TB: Well, I really didn't mean, you see, to, I just started to ask a question. In fact, they would be called defective and productive and the positive symptoms were called productive symptoms and the negative, something like defective. You know, they had different names and some people would just have the negative symptoms. Like some people would say, there are different syndrome expressions.

LG: Yes, this was really, I have to think, those studies were being done....

TB: In the late sixties?

LG: Yes and, so, the literature wasn't making that distinction and that's why I was explaining. If I wanted to, I could possible determine is there any difference? But, I haven't gotten into that right now. And I don't know, it may be productive. The trouble with some of that is, well, some of those traits might not be, this is just a thought, I think that some of those verbal behaviors might be related to personality characteristics other than schizophrenic features. For example, if somebody had a head injury or any disorder or an addiction or a lot of shock therapy, I think that might produce some of the findings that are associated with negative symptoms. I'm not sure. And, if I were to do the study, I'd want to get PET scans or MRIs to see how do these patients differentiate. Well, there had been data along that line. I think, Anders and others had those on the horizon. Apparently, there are some differences in the brain.

TB: Well, let's just, well, actually, you did make some contribution because what you, in fact it's quite a major one, because what you were, you had some findings, that level of disorganization, so there's a correlation....

LG: It's a whole classification, Social Alienation-Personal Disorganization, because that was just a name, but there are some interesting comments and phrases that people make or some comments in language that differentiates it, too.

TB: Well, that's, you know, you really....

LG: Your question is a good one. That is, I probably should have looked at and got brain scans on some of people and I wouldn't be surprised if there was difference in, but, you know, you can't do everything you want to do in an organized and funded study.

TB: Well, I really, all I.....

LG: A good question, one researcher to another.

TB: Well, you just went as far as your instruments, at that point, could go. We are, you know, MRI.

LG: We didn't have MRI then.

TB: We didn't have, even, CT was the....

LG: Right. We didn't have CT.

TB: Right, you know, this is just something.

LG: And, we certainly didn't have a PET scan.

TB: No, no, you could actually. It was just a little bit beyond a similar study.

LG: To do that.

TB: Yes, that's the other thing, but, anyway, this seems to be the major things you did in schizophrenia, you know, in the area of chronic schizophrenia, because you got them using your tests for different schizophrenic populations and you, also, cover the anxiety, because you worked with benzos, you worked with propranolol and, chemically, I think you worked with meprobamate, right?

LG: Yea.

TB: What about antidepressants? Is there anything that antidepressants in depression? Did you do any?

LG: Well, early, while I think I was still in Cincinnati, I did with imipramine.

TB: Imipramine. What did you actually do?

LG: Well, one study with imipramine, on, as a matter of fact, only milder, virtually, none depressed patients, imipramine by itself reduced the, a notable effect, the hostility levels on patients.

TB: So, what you really found in normal subjects, with imipramine...

LG: Pretty normal. And, then, there were studies with other drugs that, what were they?

TB: Amitriptyline, desipramine, reserpine?

LG: We're looking, trying to differentiate the effect of a drug, again, on personality and what they're told. And, we did studies showing that dexedrine and a mild barbiturate and a placebo--when you tell a subject--this is a drug; this is a medication that you're going to take that's going to have a stimulating effect or this is going to have a sedative effect. I was trying to differentiate the effect of what the doctor says the drug will do vs. the reaction they have, again, as measured by content analysis. And, there were, also, papers published on that research and they showed that dexedrine would tend to overcome the effect of what the doctor said. After all, there were a lot of studies then, and there still are, on how do you differentiate placebo effect from the drug effect? And how do you study that? Well, we wanted to see what effect is there in reaction to what the doctor says the drug is going to do. Well, to make a long story short, we didn't do a lot more on that, but some of that was presented, actually, at the ACNP years and years ago. Dexedrine might overcome what the doctor says. We had another scale that hasn't been described here, the Achievement Strivings scale. And we show that, even with the doctor saying this is going to make you sleepy here, and the effect of the dexedrine overcame that. It does increase Achievement Strivings; whereas, the barbiturates do not do so. And, we didn't keep on with that research, but it did show there is an effect in response to what the doctor says. No wonder these herbs (nowadays, especially) from the advertisements and so on, are having a great placebo effect, what the "expert" says. So, it has some relevance to the tie between measurement of how people feel and what the physician says.

TB: Well, so, this was, again.

LG: That's around the same time. I think I was in Cincinnati at the time.

TB: Well, this is, more or less, I suppose, the Cincinnati period, right? You have been involved in many things and, probably, you really should dedicate a lot of time to research, relatively, right?

LG: I had a practice. I was a training and supervising analyst and I had grants, but, yes, I dedicated a lot of time and that's why, as I mentioned it to you, I later took the position as Chairman at the University of California at Irvine, and there was, immediately, a very large administrative responsibility to start a residency, to get an approved residency, to get residents, to worry with all the financial problems in running a hospital. We had an emergency room that saw a thousand patients a month and to get used to the University of California. I kept my wits about me by convincing myself I had to continue to do research, so I knew who I was and what my identity was.

TB: So, all through your administrative, you know, when you were chairing the department, I would consider that, probably, the most time-consuming, administratively, right, you built a department, administratively? What proportion?

LG: I kept doing research and applying for grants.

TB: What proportion of your time would you think, you see, you spent during, I don't know, it was six, how many years were you Chairman, the founding Chairman?

LG: Oh, I would say about eleven or twelve years.

TB: Twelve. What percent time were you doing research?

LG: Twenty-five percent time.

TB: Twenty-five percent time of?

LG: Doing research.

TB: Research. How much was your practice? How much?

LG: Well, you know, just enough, because you were allowed, in that situation two half days a week to practice.

TB: So, two half days, so, really, less than twenty-five percent.

LG: Well, you don't have to do private practice. You know, you can do what you want. You can do none, if you had a ceiling, because most of the University of California pressures you to publish or perish. Well, I didn't have a problem there, but they have a very fine university system. The university is definitely a research university, whether it's humanities or physics or medicine. It rewards research and it was my type of university.

TB: So, basically, around fifty percent, a little bit more than fifty percent, administration, and twenty-five percent kind of research and the rest, practice.

LG: And, teaching.

TB: And, your teaching. Oh, and where did you put the teaching, really, how much?

LG: I know you have been a teacher in a medical school. You have more of your teaching. I tended to do more of my teaching with residents, rather than with medical students. I did give a few lectures, but I hired people. I had the right to build from scratch and get people, still all kinds. So, a lot of my teaching was with residents, and I worked up a big residency program. I had fifty or sixty residents.

TB: So, it was, mainly, with residents, rounds and this type of thing, very little classroom, right?

LG: Sometimes one on one.

TB: You were, also, supervising psychoanalysts, so you were training.

LG: Well, yes, that was everyone, analytic training analysis.

TB: I see. But, anyway, you spent, mainly, actually in teaching residents.

LG: And in research.

TB: And in research. And the research was, essentially, you had to get your research grants; so one's research was only grant dependent, whether you were able to do it or not.

LG: We are in the University of California set up and for the kind of research I was doing, you didn't always need a grant. If I was going to get, I could get a lot of residents, who wanted to do research, to get speech samples on various topics. But, in between all that, yes, I realize that if you want to do certain kinds of research and want to get a lab, you have to get big grants and I've worked for those. But, in between that, I was always able to continue to do research.

TB: Now, you already, really, had experience with EEG, at an early time of your research, right, in the early fifties, you were involved and it seems to be there was a period that you got involved in pharmacokinetics, psychopharmacology and biochemical measures in sort of for, but a little bit less than the others, and, then, you are moving to some extent, to neurophysiology, neurocerebral imaging, not even your former physiology, because you are moving as soon as brain imaging becomes possible, as soon as MRI comes about, right, or what we see?

LG: Before I got into that, there was a period of six or seven years, it had effected me, where I got a grant, a larger size of the grant, from the National Institute on Drug Abuse and this was a contract grant. You know, for seven or eight years I had to do certain jobs, but the money was just as good as anything else, and that was probably secondary to having served on federal committees, review committees, with NIDA, National Institute on Drug Abuse, or NIAAA, National Institute of Alcohol and Alcoholism or NIMH. I was on extramural review committees and I got into the project of deciding we were trying to do it and that is, I discovered that there was no uniformity across the United States on the way psychoactive drug involved are looked at, from the viewpoint of medical examiners or coroners across the United States. So there was no uniformity. And my former interest in pharmacokinetics and drug blood levels helped me towards looking at the uniformity in the way that the blood levels or the tissue levels were found by the coroners on these deceased people and the different instrumentation that was used, so the results were different. And, I got into a project, which NIDA supported for six or seven years, to develop a uniform system measuring all the variables involved in drug-involved deaths, and we had a team that developed a uniform system, made recommendations. And, say is that getting us off the topic? Well, NIDA also, gave me funds for a lab where we could check some of the findings of the coroners. And it's relevant, actually, to what we're doing today. To accommodate Oakley Ray's request for research records and notes, I have seven or eight filing cabinets of data from that study. The data with respect to those studies are stored away somewhere, and I have them all. I had to keep them, because I figured, because I've got these data from coroners and medical examiners all across the country, medical data that was supposed to be reported. Because, I wrote, then, later, you may not be familiar with it, a book, I wrote in collaboration with the head of the toxicology lab of Orange County (Louis A. Gottschalk and Robert H. Cravey. *Toxicological and Pathological Studies on Psychoactive Drug-Involved Deaths*. Davis, CA: Biomedical Publications, 1980.). And what it is, it provides the blood levels, the lung tissue levels, the other relevant tissue levels of poisoning and death due to benzodiazepines, opiates, other drugs of that sort. And it was not the purpose of this generous project grant, but I thought I have all these data and this is uniform, and it turns out that in many legal cases, it's not known whether the person died of this or that. But our book provided significant information on this matter. These people died and these were blood tissue levels found nationwide on autopsy. And it was known what drugs they took. And, I said, I didn't want to be known for this kind of research, but, on the other hand, it turned out we had these important data. We published a book on it and it's still used by a lot of coroners.

Another publication my research team and I made, at the request of the National Institute of Drug Abuse (NIDA) that funded our research on this topic was: Louis A. Gottschalk, Frederick L. McGuire, Eugene C. Dinovo, Herman Birch, Jon F. Heiser (eds.) *Guide to the Investigation and Reporting of Drug Abuse Deaths*. National Institute of Drug Abuse, ADAMHA. U.S. Dept. HEW DHEW. Publication No.(ADM)77-386, Washington D.C.: U.S. Government Printing Office, 1977, pp. 151.

TB: So, you really established a standard of what would be the measure the levels contributing to drug involved death.

LG: Well, it turns that, in legal cases, that is, there are interesting legal cases, did this person die of a morphine overdose or was this injected later, or did the person get too big a shot of insulin? There are interesting cases and if one was a mystery story writer, it could be used, but, yes, it did end up as a very important book. I don't believe the ACNP ever looked into that. Why should it, you know? The drug companies aren't so interested in those details;

however, I did get involved in that, and I don't regret it. I mean, it consumed a lot of time, lot of spare time, but it was, I think, a very worthwhile adventure.

TB: What was the name of the, you know, a famous case, was it insulin that killed him? What was it?

LG: Well, how did you know about that? Yes, there were some people that were killed by insulin.

TB: Yes.

LG: And, it can, also, be used to differentiate the cause of death. I, somehow, got involved in that issue without planning to do so.

TB: Were you involved in an insulin overdose death?

LG: No, I got involved in something else. I've been quoted, on the possible cause of Marilyn Monroe's death.

TB: I see.

LG: But, I don't want to get into that, but it was related to findings described in the book Dr. Cravey and I wrote..

TB: Later?

LG: Later, it happened. Somebody said, "Gee, I'm one of the professors of pathology". Some of the findings in that book shows that the question was, whether she overdosed or whether she was killed, say, through the mafia by an injection through her rear end of various drugs. And there were some findings that we showed had relevance to how much residue of various drugs you find in the stomach of drugs that will poison you.

TB: What was the case?

LG: Well, I don't want to go into all the details of it now. It's so far back, it's buried deep in mind, but a while back somebody wrote a book about her and the cause of her death, suggesting that it wasn't suicide.

TB: Yes, what was it?

LG: I don't remember the details. It had something to do with, if you'd taken a drug by mouth to kill yourself, you find certain residues in the stomach.

TB: Did she have the residue?

LG: Some of the books written on it and I have stayed away from that matter, rather suggested she might have been killed.

TB: Killed, I see.

LG: But, it relates to psychopharmacology in a gruesome way. However, is it relevant to what we're doing today? Well, I think the experience taught me that when somebody takes a drug, it doesn't have to go just to the brain; it gets all through the body and the liver and everything else and pathologists should look into to see what the levels are in different tissues.

TB: And, you certainly established in a large sample, you know, with different anecdotes, what would be those levels, almost regardless whether people would measure it. You gave the orientation point. And, this happened from a grant you obtained during your Psychiatry Department Chairmanship.

LG: Yes, when I was in California and we had that research grant for about six or seven years.

TB: And, you were, actually, at that point, you also had drug and alcohol institutes, right?

LG: Well, we had one.

TB: You had one.

LG: In or around that time. I think the drug and alcohol research center came later.

TB: I see.

LG: But, it certainly prepared me for this.

TB: During that time, was it during that time that you got involved with manganese and its possible contribution to violence?

LG: Well, that was much later.

TB: Much later.

LG: That was probably in the 1990's.

TB: 90's. So, we are right now in the 1980's, and in the 1980's, you, also, started with MRI, am I correct, or later?

LG: 1990's for the PET scans.

TB: PET scans, so really you didn't have as much MRI, but you moved to PET scans.

LG: PET scans because our department, probably it's unusual at that time for a single department of psychiatry, got a PET scan, probably through the efforts of William Bunney and Monte Buchsbaum. I think it's an unusual for a department to have a PET scan. It's very expensive and we got a cyclotron, and it almost drove us broke. But we have it. And usually such instrumentation is under radiology.

TB: But, it was in psychiatry.

LG: It was in psychiatry.

TB: But, Biff Bunney, it was later. But, really, this was the continuation that we are moving ahead in time than after, you know, alcohol and drug. This is the next kind of period.

LG: It was the next period.

TB: And, in the next period you are moving much into the PET scan kind of work.

LG: PET scan.

TB: PET scan. So, you left off MRI research, you did not....

LG: Well, to do PET scan and to be sure of your anatomic location, you often have to combine MRI and, so, MRI's were involved in the PET scan studies I did, often to verify the anatomical location in the change. This is the nature of PET scan. This, maybe, not always accurate, because it depends on head size and shape, so with many of those cases you did MRIs, also, but they're not featured.

TB: What was your main kind of, your major interest in PET scans? What was, you know, how would you define, how did you get involved with it? What did you try to test or what?

LG: Well, there were a number of questions I had. Dr. Monte Buchsbaum, before he left and went to Mt. Sinai Medical School in New York was certainly interested in schizophrenia and so was Dr. Bunney,

William Bunney. But, I had, you know, somewhat other interests. I was interested in that, too, and was involved in some of their research. But I was involved in such matters as, I got involved and had questions about technique, that is, when you have a PET scan, as you know, you're measuring, not just architecture of the brain and the skull, but you're measuring function. So, you're measuring what's going on in the brain of people at various times. Well, how do you stop, just because they aren't saying anything and they're in the PET scan machine, doesn't mean that they're not thinking about something. So, how do you stop them from thinking? You see, what they're thinking about might effect the PET scan. Suppose they're thinking about a love affair they had or how angry they got at a policeman arresting them. So the technique, as you know, is to have them engaged in some enterprise, right? So, the procedure is just a little bit naive. If you keep the subject engaged in doing his job and pressing a button every time something happens, a light turns on. And this procedure is presumably supposed to block out what one's random thoughts are. So, I had other questions. I thought, well, let's do some studies where you don't use this technique, you just have them be quiet and, then, report, verbally. Well, before, what's neat about the PET scans is, a person doesn't have to be thinking these things while the PET scan is being taken. Do you know that? Or maybe you're not that familiar with the PET scan procedure..

TB: No.

LG: You give an injection of the radioactive glucose and, then, have the individuals give a tape recording of their speech. Specifically, you give the injection and, then, about fifteen or twenty minutes later, you get the PET scan, because radioactive glucose takes about twenty or so many minutes to get to metabolize in the brain, different parts of the brain. So in any case, this is what we did.

And, I published a paper in Comprehensive Psychiatry, I titled: The effect of anxiety and hostility in silent mentation on cerebral glucose metabolic rate. And it showed that the subject matter that you're silently thinking about makes a difference in your cerebral glucose metabolic rates. You have these people get an injection and, then, give a speech sample of what they were thinking about, twenty minutes later, scored for anxiety and hostility. They were not told what to think about, and it demonstrated that the higher anxiety or the higher hostility, there were significant differences in their PET scans. I don't think Monte Buchsbaum was so interested in that topic. But, then, I did studies to see what parts of the brain are involved, the higher the anxiety in their dreams or the higher the hostilities of different kinds (that is, anxiety outward, anxiety inward, ambivalent hostility). And, are there differences? And, there are certainly differences than when they're awake and when they are asleep and dreaming. And we published papers in Brain Science and other journals. That was the first time that such papers were published. There were several on the differences in PET scans and the magnitude of anxiety or hostility when you are awake versus when you are asleep. There are different areas of the brain that are involved. Now, that research area is still my interest. The brain is very complicated with regards to what part is involved with different emotions and their magnitude. And, there's no other way we can study these matters at this time. And, those papers were published.

Then, I got interested in measuring hope. I had fun with that. What about hope and hopelessness and PET scans? We did the same thing and scored what somebody was silently thinking about, for hope and hopelessness. And, I got a journal—Psychiatry--that published that. There are different areas of the brain that are involved and it, certainly, makes sense, when the higher the hope versus the higher the hopelessness. So, anyway, I got into that research subject.

TB: So, really, whatever new instrumentation came, you used it.

LG: I tried to.

TB: And, basically, you raised the basic question with all your content analysis scales, the anxiety, hostility, and later on, the hope or hopelessness scales.

LG: Or the schizophrenia scale. I still have a paper that I think was ahead of its time. I had one that shows, in normal individuals, scoring them for social alienation and personal disorganization, (that's on the schizophrenic scales, but these subjects are not schizophrenics.) that the higher the scores, the more likely there's some part of the left temporal lobe involved. And it's interesting that some of the recent research on schizophrenia says, well, the left temporal lobe and frontal temporal is involved. But it's also involved in normal individuals, who are not schizophrenic, but the more, I wouldn't say social alienation and disorganization they have (though not schizophrenic), the higher their scores for glucose metabolic rates in the left temporal lobe. And, so I'm still not clear, in my mind why that seems to be so.

TB: There seems to be a continuity between this alienation and disorganization, right, in normal people as compared to more severely schizophrenic individuals.

LG: That's right.

TB: Disorganized. And, as more severe schizophrenic from the normal.

LG: Rather, than, here's a bunch of schizophrenics and here's a bunch of non-schizophrenics and they're altogether different behaviorally. Now, is it true with regards to their brain function? I don't know, but it may be, you know, if you work the statistics, you get linear continuity rather than separate, discrete characteristics.

TB: Now, most of your work was very much determined about, by your mathematical mind if you tried to sort of express things that you interpret in a mathematical kind of way.

LG: Well, you have to. Statistics has got to be used one way or the other.

TB: Well, whatever it is, you see.

LG: Or you can say, yes, I feel that science has to be on a statistical basis for your assertions to be valid; otherwise, one's assertions are a matter of faith.

TB: They are pretty much in continuing, you know, and you are, also, ambitious, essentially, you have to develop, you have to want to see, you have to have an instrument to be able to show it.

LG: Prove it.

TB: Right. Otherwise, you know, really, you've got, interestingly, almost a paradox, that at the same time you are interested in speech, you know, how the lower thing comes through.

LG: Well, I don't know why it's a paradox. You can count words; you can count numbers.

TB: Yes, but in a way, you see, you are just getting as far as it is possible to go, because you are trying to see what you can get from all of this through a free five-minute speech sample, because that is the essence, right, of your content analysis methodology.

LG: Give me five minutes or ten minutes.

TB: Five minutes, whatever it is, a standardized ambiguously elicited verbal sample without asking any questions during this five or ten minutes, or whatever it is, and it surely expresses some of the main dimensions what you would consider as important from the normal to the pathological, am I misinterpreting?

LG: You are not misinterpreting. You are right. It's not that I'm not interested in understanding other phenomena.

TB: No, no.

LG: By the way, I want to clarify that, because conversations are of great interest, you know. As I told you, I did not mention the Reagan Study, where there was a campaign debate with Mondale. I haven't gotten that yet.

TB: Maybe you should.

LG: Well, there was a political campaign debate. We have studied conversations and will publish on that soon. But it's so complicated. We're trying other studies where these conversations occur, and if you're looking at the form of speech rather than the content, you can use conversations. If I am looking at how many times that a person repeats himself, repeats, that can be useful. Well what do you mean by repeat? Counting every time there is a repetition of a word or phrase separated by no more than a word or phrase or clause, how often does a person repeat himself. A word, phrase or clause, separated by no more than a word, phrase or clause, it doesn't matter what you say, you can just look at that. Well, those issues and those facts and those data turn out to be important in older people or people that They have brain injury. They are more repetitious, no question about it, or, but it's also related to age. If you've got little kids, they often repeat themselves. But, then, it's also sometimes related to the vocation of the person. If you get a clergyman or politician, they will say, "I tell you, I tell you that we have to defeat," and they repeat themselves for emphasis. So, you do have to look at that, you know, the ministers and the clergy and the rabbis, do often repeat themselves for emphasis. But, I just want to point that out that the whole system can apply to, that we've developed, to conversation, but, then, you have to watch the research design or verbal text. You can say, what do you mean, verbal text? Well, there are people that use our method, and we published on that, and they want to compare and look at the documents that were written before the French Revolution and whether there was an increasing amount, now, this is in French, of hostility to the royalty. So, you know, they're just using documents. Are there people that have gotten into this? Somebody's asked, is there more hope in the New York Times, different times and different words if you just take the front page? You see, content analysis is getting more and more popular and people are looking at text, and we can look at the TV stories, I mean, right now, with this Kosovo thing, you know, is there more about war, battle, illness?

And, so, anyway, the whole system, can it be applied to verbal text?

TB: You started to say, you see, that the Reagan Study or Reagan Story, I don't know what, you know, if you could just continue on that them.

LG: Yes, I'll come back to that. I'm glad you do that. I'm wandering away some, but I am doing that to provide an example of the application of the content analysis measure as a detector of cognitive impairment. About 1984, I was consulted by Gannett Publications from Washington, D.C., that I had been recommended to them by the American Psychiatric Association in Washington, D.C., that I had a content analysis measure derived from speech and would I collaborate with them. Would I measure the relative cognitive impairment in the debaters, specifically of Reagan and Mondale, in their debates? So, I said, "Alright". They'd send me the tapes and the video. I reflected that in a political debate the debater could not read a prewritten script; he had to be spontaneous and somewhat unprepared. And, I did number one of the debate, then number two. I looked at that, myself, at that time. I didn't have a computer program to do this, and I noted that when Reagan didn't have a script, he had to freelance; he had to be spontaneous. And, my goodness! His scores on scorable content analysis items for cognitive impairment were significantly higher than Mondale's. What I used as another control was the interviewers themselves, since they were neutral. I mean, they asked questions, and they could show cognitive problems. In this case, it wasn't five-minute samples. So, I told Gannett Publications what I had found, but I would like to get the earlier debates of Reagan with Carter, four years earlier. And, they got those and looking at those data, and the content in the cognitive impairment scale, Reagan didn't look as bad as he did four years later debating Mondale.

And, I said, "Oh, oh, should we publish anything?" Well, now, this is before the election and I don't think I'll tell the story that I'd told you earlier, but I thought it was kind of amusing because Dr. Bunney didn't think we should publish it, or I should publish it. And, he was worried that, that might bias the National Institutes of Health, not worrying about our research. Oh, I'll tell the story. So, I asked the Dean of the College of Medicine, at that time. What should I ask the Dean, because it involves our school. And, so, I asked Dean, Stanley van den Noort. He said, "How did it come out, really?" I said, "Well, Reagan didn't look that good." He said, "Publish it!" Well, I said, "Stanley, you're a Democrat." "You bet." So, I told Bunney about this and he said, "Oh, well, he's biased. Ask the Chancellor." And the Chancellor, at that time, was Jack Peltason, a political scientist and economist, and a guy that I respected and I asked him about it. He said, "Well, I don't know much about content analysis, but was it scientific and valid? I said it was. He said, "Publish it." But, I decided not to publish it right away, because I thought, well, there are these criticisms of people in the American Psychiatric Association, current at that time. Some psychiatrists said something psychiatrically negative about Goldwater without ever interviewing him. But, at least, in my case, I had verbal data and, so, I waited till after the presidential election. I asked a colleague of mine in the school of business, with whom I was on a University of California Promotions Committee, could he recommend a top rate non-psychiatric publication. He suggested Public Administration Review published out of Washington, D.C. He said, send it there, I think, they'll be glad, if it's a good paper they'll publish it. And, it had a lot of statistics in it, and they published it. And, that was published in 1988, I think. Well, when I was scored on that one, there were criticisms of it and some of them were, oh, this psychiatric gobbledy goop, this guy doesn't know what he's talking about, so I don't believe it. But, we know what happened to President Ronald Reagan, later—he developed Alzheimer's disease. And, I do know that the cognitive impairment scales are very sensitive as well as valid. They can pick up, (I kid about it sometimes, but it wouldn't be a bad idea to try it on the pilot of your airplane to be sure to test him, because it will even show up, whether somebody is on an antihistamine, alcohol, or benzodiazepine. It's very sensitive.

TB: No, it's, obviously so; this makes a case, you know, for sensitivity. And it looks like it is, I don't know, much more sensitive than any kind of psychiatric assessments.

LG: Well, very, very simple and easy to get and I noticed somebody, recently, was in the news. Somebody got a test, picked up early Alzheimer's. You give thirty things for a person to remember, objects maybe, light, table and an ordinary person can pick fifteen, but an early Alzheimer's can only get about seven or eight. And, my test will do the same, pick it up. I did, on the last study, you know, get onto that.

TB: Well, this test is really, probably, your most important contribution, in general, right? Well, let me sort of pick it up from this. What would you consider your most important contribution within psychopharmacology? You talked, actually, about a couple like thioridazine. What would you consider your most important single contribution within the field of psychopharmacology?

LG: That's like asking a guy, well, you've got four children or six children, which one do you like the best? And, I care about all of them. I don't know what that is. Now, you're asking me to be objective. I think my contributions in the general field of neuropsychopharmacology are good and original. I think my contributions to the measurement of neurobiological and psychobiological states, to the now computerized content of natural language or verbal text, is very important. I think the neurobiological studies with PET scan, I mean, or brain imaging are important. I think, to me, they're all my children and they're equally important. Now, somebody else might think, you may know ten years from now. Well, that was old stuff. It's sometimes in the midst of doing these things, it's hard to realize.

TB: I understand.

LG: I'm just telling how I feel about your question. Well, you might think that this guy is pretty narcissistic; he loves all his children, but I just think they're all relevant and I can't. I'm not a good judge. Time, alone, will tell.

TB: Yes, but at this point, you see, you really would like the verbal content of speech analysis, that's what you really feel that people should use more extensively, am I correct?

LG: I don't use the word, "should," for others, because, now, they say this guy sounds like a controlling person.

TB: I'm not saying should, but you would.

LG: No, I'm getting a growing conviction that it's a very sensitive, useful measure and, in time, it might turn out to be even better and useful for society.

TB: Now, you seem to be involved in so many areas. We really touched on, besides psychopharmacology and neurobiology, you see, in all different ways. Is there any other areas completely, something that you haven't covered at all, up to this point, that you...

LG: In science?

TB: In science or in other work. You really feel you made kind of?

LG: I like to do art; but I'm an amateur artist. I do a little water color, but, no, I'm trying, now, to write a, I'm in the process of writing. I have written a novel. It was semi successful, but I'm writing a documentary on my personal experiences in World War II, on seeing maybe thousands of neuropsychiatric cases, and I've had a criticism of it from Simon Schuster. They think it's too academic, and I'm trying to rewrite it and elaborate, and I'm having fun with that. Now, is that going to be an important contribution? No, but in these times, I don't think, well, most times, the neuropsychiatric casualties in a war are in conflict with patriotism or deemphasized. It seems alright to get a Purple Heart or to have been injured in the military and you get honors. Or it seems alright if you went AWOL or you got drunk or you told an officer off, but, at least that's manly. And, there's a certain amount of honor in being a Robin Hood, but neuropsychiatric casualties, and what they effect? The effect is suppressed. And, I saw, we each had a large caseload at that hospital, the United Public Health Service Hospital, you know, one hundred ten or one hundred twenty cases, plus those World War I cases (N=300+) I acquired that were transferred from St. Elizabeth's Hospital in Washington, D.C. And I think that's just scratching the surface. There are many people that served, and guys and gals that served in the military were traumatized. They didn't have a nervous breakdown, but it effected them; it scarred them, and it has long-term adverse effects. Because I see them, subsequently, through the Veterans Administration. It has effects on their physical health and their mental health. Some of them die younger. And, so, I'm into that right now.

TB: That's what you're rewriting right now?

LG: Yes, I'm rewriting it and trying to make a good point. (My book, World War II. Neuropsychiatric Casualties. Out of Sight. Out of Mind was published by Nova Science Publishers, Inc.: New York, in 2004. Its sales have been good.)

TB: You had been involved in social kind of prospects. We didn't talk anything, you had, really, an appointment as Professor of Sociology.

LG: Yes, that was Social Science.

TB: Social Science, yes. Is there anything special you would of like to sort put on the record, what you did?

LG: Well, I think that psychiatry is not just biological science, but it involves a person's behavior and society, I think during the time I was more active in the Social Science division, but I think I did, in retrospect, a landmark study and that is The Effect of Sensory Overload on Behavior. And, I had a graduate student (Daniel E. Bates), I think it was in Social Science during that period of time, and he had a similar interest. And he and I planned together, we had built, a dome like structure, I suppose ten feet in diameter at the bottom, and going upward and the a subject was supposed to lie down on the floor in there and we had a Technicolor film made, a movie of music and odd colors. And we put the subject in that dome-like structure, lying down, and looking upwards, and the whole film was projected up into the ceiling of that dome. And we got verbal samples before and after the sensory overload experience. And, there was no question, after being in that for fifteen minutes and their verbal samples before and after the sensory overload experience, they showed significant elevation of that schizophrenic scale, significant elevations. And, that was published (Louis A. Gottschalk, John L. Haer, Daniel E. Bates. Effect of Sensory Overload on psychological state. *Mental Health Digest*. 5:29-31, 1973). Well, a lot has been made of that since, to some extent. It's regarded now as a form of gate-ing, that there are some people that are able to compartmentalize events and perceptual experiences of that sort and shut things out. And, we had some other tests, the Rod and Frame tests. I don't know if you're familiar with that. Those are various tests that indicate whether people are influenced in their perception of events. Are they influenced some by the frame in which a rod is placed, or are they just looking at the rod? Are they influenced a lot by the surroundings of an event? And, we found that people that have, this is a standard test, people that are influenced a lot by the surroundings are more susceptible to this extrasensory overload. And we proved that with this measure. Now, that came out of the Social Science division, because I was working with a graduate student in there. And a lot of people have asked me, since, do we have that dome-like structure that we built and do I have the movie. I think I probably still have the movie. But, the relevance, I think that's still relevant for those people and you can see in the Archives at General Psychiatry, it's often in there, about this whole concept of gate-ing. Does a schizophrenic have not such good gaiting, cutting out stuff? Are they hypersensitive? Now, this was on a bunch of normal students.

TB: It seems to be, then, you have to continue them, right? But, what you are saying is the ones who are more sensitive, right?

LG: Right, whether genetic or some other way. In this case, there's a guy, a friend of mine (Prof. J. Christian Gillin, also a member of ACNP) in San Diego, who made a lot of that study. He used a lot of that idea and findings in his own research. I think there is something to this gate-ing proposition.

TB: So, you really, did do some interesting work in Social Science. What about Ecology, because you did some work in Ecology?

LG: Social Ecology.

TB: Social Ecology, what did you do?

LG: Well, I think they liked me. They didn't pay any salary. That shows the effect of ecology; it's like the study I was talking about, drug-related deaths. Out of those studies, we looked at a suicide, the effect on environment in suicide, or drug overdose. So, all that was relevant. I wrote a paper that was published and it's in one of the books, What About Interrogation? Can somebody lie under interrogation or not? This is looking at, what about the environment, the effect of environment on speech? But, usually, you and I don't get involved in interrogation. That's not our field. But, I got involved in that and did some review of the literature on that subject and I wrote on it. And, I was asked, actually, by the military to help on that, too. I suppose, some of our soldiers get captured by the Koreans, in those wars. And they are put under their stressful interview, possibly torture, (Dr. Jolly West, I don't know whether you knew him; he was Department Chair of UCLA, and was interested in the subject.) and effects of interrogation, and what do you do in a situation?

TB: It was West, wasn't it?

LG: Jolly West.

TB: Jolly West.

LG: And, out of the studies that I did, but it was mostly literature (I don't do that type of interrogation), but it's relevant, if you get captured (and, I passed my ideas on to the military). I recommended taking LSD or something like that, act crazy, because they're not going to interrogate you, if they think you're crazy because they will believe that your information is not reliable. If they kill you, that's against the law. But, you know, if you're captured, don't let them put you through all this kind of torture. And, as far as I know, my suggestions have has been followed, to some extent. But, you say, what has that got to do with Social Ecology? Well, it has the effect of the environment on how much somebody will share?

TB: Now, it happens to be that I worked with you on Cameron, you know, who had been involved in somewhat similar kind of report.). Do you remember Cameron?

LG: Oh, from Canada.

TB: Canada. Allan Memorial Institute, Montreal, and, you know, we had been involved in sensory isolation and I was, really, the resident, who was working with Cameron, or psychic driving, but, you know, anyway, I'm quite familiar with the kind of work that you had, we're talking about. There are a couple of books written. Let's go back for a second just to ask you a simple, very simple question. Again, back into the psychopharmacology, we have covered almost everything, really. I mean, it's impossible to cover everything, but we touched on all of the different aspects.

LG: Well, it would be taking LSD to be crazy, so persons won't pay attention to you. Is that related to psychopharmacology and an unusual aspect?

TB: Have you been involved in the chemical development of any psychotropic drugs? I do know that you did some very early work with perphenazine, because you did it, did you not?

LG: No, no, on the clinical development. But no I would consider being involved in a putative anti-anxiety drug and the original test of it is involved. But it was not at the manufacturing level. It's, yes, a number of those early studies on the benzodiazepines was, was this diazepam or triazolame or any of these other drugs, do they really have anti-anxiety, action? And, in those times, I was collaborating with the head of pharmacology (a Professor Henry Elliott, M.D., Ph.D.); we did these studies and they were used by the drug company to decide to market these psychoactive drugs. That was early, but that was only at that level.

TB: That was only that time.

LG: Not developing in a laboratory.

TB: You seem to be very active in so many levels. Now, have you ever been active in regulations, you know, have you contributed to any kind of regulation, which is related to drugs or mental health?

LG: I don't know exactly what you mean by regulations. I think, in the drug abuse.

TB: Drug abuse or in any kind of....

LG: Well, I don't know, you mean, the legal regulations?

TB: Regulations, legal, right. Legal aspect sort of....

LG: Well, I don't know, you see. This current research that I have been doing with NIDA, National Institute on Drug Abuse, they've asked for software that will detect and measure cognitive impairment in drug-abusing patients and they're continually, primarily, interested in illegal drugs and that's turned out to be positive. And we're continuing to do those studies, further.

At one end, I mean, I haven't told, but I wouldn't be surprised if NIDA or the federal government might use that with respect to regulations, early detection. I don't know what they want to do with that. Now, that would be one area. Have there been others on regulation? Well, when I was in research, I was a clinician at the United States Public Health Service Hospital, narcotic hospital, and there, I was a practitioner, even though, I was there in a military role, they still had that hospital open for voluntary and involuntary admissions, who were addicts. And, either way. The government would take voluntary admissions and not charge them. I was regularly involved there, in a different role. But, why would voluntary patients come there? Well, most of the time it turned out they were on high doses of a morphine or a derivative, and they wanted to get on lower doses so it would be cheaper for them. And, we still had to take them in. Well, is that regulation? Yes, because some of those patients were there because they smoked marijuana, and they had to be there legally. And, probably, working in there, probably, contributed to my deciding never to smoke marijuana; although, some great musicians smoke it. And, then, another study I did on regulation, I haven't mentioned that. It's a kind of psychopharmacologic study at the VA. There was a colleague there, a cardiologist, that thought that there was some evidence that marijuana smoking may relieve angina and I got involved with him, studying that. We used marijuana, smoking marijuana and placebo-marijuana, and we found out that if you put these patients in the VA, who have angina, on a treadmill on a placebo-marijuana, they don't do so well. Then, you put them on real marijuana and they go for a helluva long time on the treadmill. But, we also got simultaneous the echocardiograms and the ones who kept going for a long time, their echocardiograms were terrible. So, we learned, now, is that a legal thing? Well, we learned that marijuana is a good but it disconnects the brain from cardiac and bodily function. And, it might be good, you know, we didn't say that, but it might be good for people that are dying or something. But, I mean, to keep in touch with what's happening to your body, it minimized or delimited the pain reaction they had, but they could die. So, that's another area.

TB: Again, an important study.

LG: Study.

TB: Right.

LG: You would say, well, that was psychosomatic, yes. We, also, got verbal samples on those people that show when they were on marijuana smoking, they had significantly higher social alienation personal disorder and cognitive impairment, you know.

So, it's like somebody that takes a little booze. They may feel good, but, you know, I wouldn't trust them as much to know, to take an exam in math or something like that. There probably are times when you and I have to undergo an operation or something of that sort to be anesthetized, you know, but probably not for just all therapeutic reasons. Pain killers probably work the same way, anesthetize a little bit of our brain.

TB: Well, that's actually a very nice end, you know. We really, I think we covered more or less with that subject. If there is something you really would to add, anything you....

LG: Well, yes, only one other thing, it doesn't seem, yes, it's related some. These later studies, in that earlier CV, we did find, we had done some studies on stuttering and that risperidone reduces the severity of stuttering. But, in the same papers that we're publishing, they're impressing that (inaudible).

TB: I'd say, new, that's one of the most recent, right?

LG: Yes, but it's likely, the sensitive test we have, that stutterers do have a certain type of cognitive impairment. They might be brilliant in some areas and they could be. And the stuttering doesn't interfere with their IQ, but they do have some kind of cognitive function impairment, and there's PET scan studies that support that. I think that should be reported.

TB: And, this really your last paper?

LG: No, the last paper I'm trying to get a research study grant. This is on The Detection of Cognitive Impairment from Verbal Samples and eventually being able to do this from voice recognition, so the speech doesn't have to be typed and you have to, laboriously, go through typing it up. But it can be directly done by some of the new techniques and technology and voice recognition.

TB: So, again, your last paper is integrating a new technique to use it, to forward, actually, to speed things up and make it easier, more accessible.

LG: Right.

TB: I think we, more or less, covered everything. I just would like to thank you very much for this very interesting kind of few hours. I think the information you gave us is very educational. It's very important.

LG: It's been enjoyable talking to you.

TB: Very nice to talk to you.

LG: About one of my favorite subjects.

TB: Thank you. Thank you very much.

INDEX

A

B

C

D

E

F

G

H

I

J

K

L

Q

R

S

W

X

Y